T0340720

Arthropod-borne Infectious Diseases of the Dog and Cat

Susan E Shaw

BVSc(Hons) MSc DipACVIM DipECVIM FACVSc MRCVS
Senior Lecturer in Veterinary Dermatology and Applied Immunology
School of Clinical Veterinary Science
University of Bristol
Langford, Bristol, UK

Michael J Day

BSc BVMS(Hons) PhD DiplECVP FASM FRCPath FRCVS
Professor of Veterinary Pathology
School of Clinical Veterinary Science
University of Bristol
Langford, Bristol, UK

LIPPINCOTT WILLIAMS & WILKINS
A **Wolters Kluwer** Company

Philadelphia • Baltimore • New York • London
Buenos Aires • Hong Kong • Sydney • Tokyo

Dedication

To all colleagues and students who have as much enthusiasm
for this subject as I do (SES)

To Lara, Christopher and Natalie (MJD)

First published in the United States of America in 2005 by
Lippincott, Williams & Wilkins, 351 Camden Street, Baltimore, MD 21201

ISBN 0-7817-9014-X

Copyright © 2005 Manson Publishing Ltd, London, UK

A CIP catalog record for this book is available from the publisher.

For full details of all Manson Publishing Ltd titles please write to:
73 Corringham Road, London NW11 7DL, UK
www.mansonpublishing.com

Commissioning editor: Jill Northcott
Project manager: Paul Bennett
Copy-editor: Peter Beynon
Designer: Replika Press Pvt Ltd, India
Colour reproduction: Tenon & Polert Colour Scanning Ltd, Hong Kong
Printed by: Grafos SA, Barcelona, Spain

Contents

Preface

The study of arthropod-borne infectious disease in companion animals is developing rapidly. For example, new species and subspecies of *Babesia* affecting dogs and cats are being characterized as this book is being written. In addition, it is highly likely that the role of arthropods in the transmission of other important canine and feline diseases will be confirmed. This is particularly the case with the haemoplasmas (previously *Haemobartonella* species) of dogs and cats, where investigation of transmission by *Ctenocephalides felis* (the cat flea) is the subject of current intensive research.

With this background, we set out to produce a text that would collect together the important information related to the arthropod-borne infectious diseases of companion animals. Our objectives in producing this book were:

To provide veterinary surgeons with comprehensive information on clinical presentation, pathogenesis, diagnosis, treatment, control and zoonotic implications of the major arthropod-transmitted diseases of dogs and cats (Chapters 5 to 13).

- To provide additional information in the same text on relevant aspects of the biology of the arthropod vectors and their wildlife host species. It is hoped this will encourage greater understanding of the challenges required in controlling these infections as well as an appreciation of the biological complexities involved in their maintenance (Chapters 1 and 2).
- To provide additional information in the same text on the immunological interactions between arthropod-borne pathogens, their vectors and the companion animal hosts (Chapter 3). Immune–mediated disease is a hallmark of infection with this specific group of pathogens, and it is hoped that Chapter 3 will provide veterinary surgeons with a basis for understanding and interpreting the clinical and laboratory evidence for this in cases with suspected arthropod-borne disease. In addition, appreciation of this complex interaction provides a platform for understanding both the difficulties involved in the development of traditional vaccines for this group of infections and the development of novel immunomodulatory approaches to treatment.

- To provide more detailed information in the same text on the expanding array of diagnostic techniques routinely available to veterinary surgeons dealing with these diseases (Chapter 4). Arthropod-transmitted diseases provide a real diagnostic challenge. Many tests are available for the same disease, using different technologies and with differing sensitivities and specificities. Tests for exposure to infection, such as antibody-based serology, provide different information from those designed to identify active infection (PCR-based methods). Both sets of information may be useful in difficult cases and Chapter 4 has been written to enable veterinary practitioners to better understand the laboratory basis for the results they receive.

Arthropod-Borne Infectious Diseases of the Dog and Cat is a project that has arisen from the clinical, laboratory diagnostic and research interests of the editors in this rapidly developing field of veterinary medicine. Over a number of years we have met and collaborated with many veterinarians and scientists active in this field who have become valued colleagues and friends. Many of these have contributed the chapters, illustrations or data that form this book. To these contributors we are exceedingly grateful for your excellent reviews and prompt responses to questions or proofreading. Your enthusiasm and rigorous scientific input has helped us to produce a text of which we can all be proud.

We must also acknowledge the superb support from Manson Publishing for this project. The book was born from early discussions with Jill Northcott and we are grateful for her support and gentle cajoling throughout. Michael Manson has been characteristically supportive and it has been a pleasure to work with him. We are very pleased to be able to thank the production team headed by Paul Bennett, and the expert and detailed copyediting provided by Peter Beynon. The hand-drawn sketches produced by individual contributors have been expertly rendered into a uniform style by Cactus Design and Illustration.

We hope this book will prove an informative and practical resource to practising veterinarians who deal with this fascinating group of diseases.

Susan Shaw and Michael Day

Contributors

Gad Baneth DVM PhD DiplECVCP
School of Veterinary Medicine
Hebrew University
Rehovot, Israel

Anneli Björsdorff DVM PhD
Department of Clinical Microbiology
Kalmar County Hospital
Kalmar, Sweden

Malcolm Bennett BVSc PhD FRCPath MRCVS
Department of Veterinary Pathology
University of Liverpool
Neston, United Kingdom

Richard J Birtles BSc(Hons) PhD
Centre for Comparative Infectious Diseases
University of Liverpool
Neston, United Kingdom

Kevin Bown BSc(Hons) MRes PhD
Department of Veterinary Pathology
University of Liverpool
Neston, United Kingdom

Michael J Day BSc BVMS(Hons) PhD DiplECVP FASM
FRCPath FRCVS
School of Clinical Veterinary Science
University of Bristol
Langford, United Kingdom

Luca Ferasin DVM PhD CertVC DipECVIM-CA
(Cardiology) MRCVS
School of Clinical Veterinary Science
University of Bristol
Langford, United Kingdom

Craig E Greene DVM MS DipACVIM(Internal Medicine
and Neurology)
Department of Infectious Disease
College of Veterinary Medicine
University of Georgia
Athens, United States of America

Shimon Harrus DVM PhD DiplECVCP
School of Veterinary Medicine
Hebrew University
Rehovot, Israel

K Emil Hovius DVM MSc PhD
Companion Animal Hospital 't Heike
Veldhoven, The Netherlands

Peter J Irwin BVetMed PhD FACVSc MRCVS
School of Veterinary and Biomedical Sciences
Murdoch University
Murdoch, Western Australia

Martin J Kenny BSc PhD
School of Clinical Veterinary Science
University of Bristol
Langford, United Kingdom

David Harmon Knight DVM DipACVIM(Cardiology) (decd)
Veterinary Hospital
University of Pennsylvania
Philadelphia, United States of America

Kieren Pitts BSc MSc PhD
School of Biological Sciences
University of Bristol
Bristol, United Kingdom

Xavier Roura DVM PhD DipECVIM-CA
Servei de Medicina Interna
Hospital Clínic Veterinari
Universitat Autònoma de Barcelona
Bellaterra, Spain.

Susan E Shaw BVSc(Hons) MSc DipACVIM DipECVIM
FACVSc MRCVS
School of Clinical Veterinary Science
University of Bristol
Langford, United Kingdom

Nancy A Vincent-Johnson DVM MS DipACVIM DipACVPM
Lieutenant Colonel, U.S. Army Veterinary Corps
Commander, National Capital District Veterinary Command
Fort Belvoir, United States of America

Richard Wall BSc MBA PhD
School of Biological Sciences
University of Bristol
Bristol, United Kingdom

Trevor Waner BVSc PhD DipECLAM
Israel Institute for Biological Research
Ness Ziona, Israel

Abbreviations

ACA   acrodermatitis chronica atrophicans
AIDS   acquired immune deficiency syndrome
ALP   alkaline phosphatase
ALT   alanine aminotransferase
AMP   adenosine monophosphate
ANA   antinuclear antibody
APC   antigen presenting cell
APTT   activated partial thromboplastin time
ARDS   adult respiratory distress syndrome
ATIII   antithrombin III
BSK   Barbour–Stoenner–Kelly (medium)
CFUs   colony forming units
CK   creatine kinase
CME   canine monocytic ehrlichiosis
CNS   central nervous system
CSD   cat scratch disease
DEC   diethylcarbamazine citrate
DIC   disseminated intravascular coagulation
DNA   deoxyribonucleic acid
DTH   delayed type hypersensitivity
EM   erythema migrans
ERIC   enterobacterial repetitive intergenic consensus
FAT   fluorescent antibody test
FDP   fibrin degradation products
FeLV   feline leukaemia virus
FIV   feline immunodeficiency virus
FML   fucose mannose ligand
GGT   gamma glutamyl transferase
gp   glycoprotein
HAI   *Hepatazoon americanum* infection
HCI   *Hepatazoon canis* infection
HGE   human granulocytic ehrlichiosis
HIV   human immunodeficiency virus
HME   human monocytic ehrlichiosis
HWD   heartworm disease
IFA   immunofluorescent assay
IFAT   indirect fluorescent antibody test
Ig   immunoglobulin (IgA, IgG, etc)
kDa   kilodaltons
LPS   lipopolysaccharide
MHC   major histocompatability complex
Micro-IF microimmunofluorescence (test)
MLST   multilocus sequence typing
MPGM   membranoproliferative glomerulonephritis
NSAID   non-steroidal anti-inflammatory drug
OspA/B/C outer surface protein A/B/C
PACAP   pituitary adenylate cyclase-activating polypeptide

PAMPs   pathogen-associated molecular patterns
PBL   peripheral blood lymphocytes
PCR   polymerase chain reaction
PCV   packed cell volume
PDGF   platelet-derived growth factor
PFGE   pulsed field gel electrophoresis
PLN   protein losing nephropathy
PT   prothrombin time
PTE   pulmonary thromboembolism
RAPD   random amplification of polymorphic DNA
RH   relative humidity
RIM   rapid immunomigration
RMSF   Rocky Mountain spotted fever
RNA   ribonucleic acid
R_O reproductive rate
SDS-PAGE sodium dodecyl sulphate polyacrylamide gel electrophoresis
SFG   spotted fever group
SGE   salivary gland extract
SPF   specific pathogen-free
TBEV   tick-borne encephalitis virus
TCP   trimethoprim-sulphadiazine, clindamycin and pyrimethamine (therapy)
Th   T helper (cell)
TP   total protein
WHO   World Health Organization
WNV   West Nile virus
WS   Warthin–Starry (stain)
ZVL   zoonotic visceral leishmaniosis

Introduction
Susan Shaw and Michael Day

The arthropod-borne infectious diseases that are the subject of this book have received much attention in both human and veterinary medicine in recent years. This interest is part of a more general focus on infectious disease, and the realization that the pattern and prevalence of infection, either locally or globally, change over time. There are several reasons why these changes occur:

- Emergence of new diseases caused by novel pathogens that appear following adaptation of existing pathogenic organisms and, less commonly, by genetic mutation. Epidemiological analysis has defined the likely 'profile' of emerging human pathogens and suggested that viruses are more likely to be considered emergent pathogens than bacteria, protozoa or fungi. Moreover, vector-transmitted pathogens are more likely to be regarded as emergent than those transmitted by direct or environmental contact (*Table 1*).
- Emergence of a disease in a new geographical area. Until 1999, West Nile virus had never been documented in the western hemisphere, although it was well established in the human, bird and vertebrate populations of Europe, Africa, western Asia and the Middle East. Since its first appearance in the eastern USA, West Nile virus has become established in the bird and mosquito populations of most of the USA. The factors involved in the introduction of West Nile virus into North America are incompletely understood. The viral genotype is most closely related to those found in the Middle East, and its introduction from this area by infected humans, vectors and/or birds has been suggested.
- Re-emergence of a previously controlled disease. A combination of decreased resources, political and social factors and complacency has led to the re-emergence of vector-transmitted diseases in the last ten years. Decreased control of vector populations resulting from the withdrawal of dichlorodiphenyltrichlorethane (DDT) for environmental reasons has compromised the control of mosquito populations and thus of malaria. Breakdown in public health infrastructure in developing countries has compromised vaccination programmes for diseases such as yellow fever. In addition, the increasing prevalence of human immunodeficiency virus (HIV) infection in areas endemic for vector-borne diseases has resulted in increased susceptibility to leishmaniosis and its emergence as a major global zoonosis. Increased travel, global travel, urbanization and population density are all playing a role in disease re-emergence.

Table 1 Profile of an emerging human pathogen.

The most likely emergent human pathogen would be:
- An RNA virus.
- Zoonotic, with a broad reservoir-host range.
- Vector transmitted, especially by biting flies that feed on multiple host species.
- Able to use a cell receptor that is conserved across host species.
- Potentially transmissible between humans (such transmission is currently rare).
- Found in areas undergoing ecological, demographic or social change.

(After Woolhouse MEJ (2002) *Trends in Microbiology* **10**, S3–S7)

Some infectious diseases may appear to be emerging simply because the pathogen involved has been recently recognized and characterized. Technical improvements and wider availability of sensitive diagnostic methodology, such as polymerase chain reaction (PCR) analysis, have enabled identification of pathogens that are not amenable to traditional methods of diagnosis such as microbial culture. Linked to this, greater recognition of such infections by improved training of diagnosticians, and the specific interests of researchers, is likely to play a role.

All of the general principles involved in the emergence of infectious diseases mentioned above are important in the mounting significance of arthropod-borne infections in companion animals. Indeed, the increasing requests for information about these infections from veterinary surgeons now required to deal with them for the first time, was the major impetus for the production of this book. However, there are specific factors that have been or may be implicated in the geographical spread of arthropod-borne infections of companion animals. They will be discussed in greater detail in the chapters that follow, but are introduced here.

Of perhaps greatest significance in the emergence of companion animal arthropod-transmitted infections is increased movement of dogs and cats over long distances and through different bioclimatic zones. The introduction and establishment of *Ehrlichia canis* and *Babesia gibsoni* in certain areas of the USA has been related to the relocation of infected military dogs. Dogs travelling from northern European countries to Mediterranean areas for vacations with their owners have been incriminated in the establishment of *E. canis* infection and the vector of this pathogen, *Rhipicephalus sanguineus*, in Germany. Frequency and ease of canine travel is also implicated in the relatively rapid dissemination of *Leishmania infantum* infection in foxhounds from foci in the eastern USA.

The traditional barrier of companion animal quarantine is being phased out between many countries and, within Europe, simplification of requirements for pet animal movement across borders is one part of the current political move towards greater integration. In the UK, abolition of quarantine for animals entering from numerous other countries has resulted in diseases previously considered exotic to the country (e.g. monocytic ehrlichiosis, babesiosis) being seen by veterinary practitioners for the first time in non-quarantined animals.

The introduction of infected animals into non-endemic areas may be associated with the development of non-traditional modes of transmission. In both Australia and the USA, transmission of *B. gibsoni* by biting has been incriminated in the sudden appearance of infection in dog breeds used for fighting. In the UK, alternative arthropod vectors may be involved in the transmission of *Leishmania infantum* from infected imported to non-travelled dogs in the absence of the usual sandfly vectors. Finally, as in humans, the spread of infection through blood transfusions by-passing the vector can occur, particularly where no exposure history is available for donors.

The threat of increased geographical extension of these diseases and the establishment of new areas of endemnicity is a real one. The well-documented effect of climate change means that environments that were traditionally unsuited for the maintenance of particular arthropod vectors may become so in the near future. Additionally, within existing endemic areas, climatic change may lead to enhancement or extended periods of transmission of vector-borne disease. The recent northerly spread of tick-borne encephalitis in Scandinavia has been directly related to the effect of increased temperatures on tick distribution and survival.

The increasing need for arable/pasture land and housing has led to increased contact of both humans and companion animals with vectors and wildlife reservoirs of arthropod-borne infections. Dogs in particular are commonly involved with sporting and leisure activities in environments conducive to arthropod exposure. A recent study examining the effect of clearing forest for housing developments showed that where relatively small areas of forest (under two hectares) were left, the density of small rodent species and the ticks that feed on them increases dramatically. This effect is secondary to the loss of larger predator species within the small forest plots. A similar effect has been suggested for mosquito populations within cleared Amazonian rainforest.

Although not a 'natural' means of increased prevalence of arthropod-borne infectious disease, it is clear that a number of the infectious agents described within this book are potential candidates for spread via bioterrorism. There has been much discussion within the veterinary profession of the likely role of veterinary surgeons in identifying possible outbreaks of infection that may be spread to the animal and human population in this manner.

1 Arthropod vectors of infectious disease: biology and control

Richard Wall and Kieren Pitts

INTRODUCTION

The blood-feeding behaviour of a wide range of arthropods makes them important vectors of infectious disease in cats and dogs. This chapter discusses the biology of the haematophagous arthropods most relevant to transmission of disease in companion animals.

TICKS

Ticks are obligate, blood-feeding ectoparasites, closely related to mites. They form a relatively small order of only about 800 species in the subclass Acari. However, they are one of the most important groups of arthropod disease vectors. A single family of ticks, the Ixodidae (known as the hard ticks), and in particular species of *Rhipicephalus*, *Ixodes* and *Dermacentor*, are of paramount importance as vectors of disease for dogs and cats, since they may transmit a range of viral, bacterial and protozoan pathogens. A second family of ticks, the Argasidae (the soft ticks), are parasites primarily of birds, bats and reptiles and will not be discussed here.

The major tick species known to be of importance in transmitting disease to dogs and cats are summarized in *Table 2*. The brown dog tick *Rhipicephalus sanguineus* is one of the most widely distributed species of ticks found worldwide. Its primary host is the dog, and all life-cycle stages may feed on this host. They often infest kennels and domestic premises, where feeding activity may occur all year round. Throughout much of northern Europe and Asia, the most common species of tick infesting dogs and cats is the sheep tick, *Ixodes ricinus*. It is commonly found in pastures and mixed woodland, where the larval and nymphal stages feed primarily on small mammals and ground-nesting birds and the adult stages on deer or

Table 2 Main tick species known to transmit pathogens to dogs and cats.

Family	Subfamily	Genera	Key species	Distribution
Ixodidae	Ixodinae (Prostriata)	*Ixodes*	I. ricinus (sheep, deer tick),	Europe
			I. hexagonus (hedgehog tick)	Europe and north-west Africa
			I. scapularis (black-legged tick)	Eastern North America
			I. pacificus (Western black-legged tick)	Western North America
			I. persulcatus (Taiga tick)	Northeastern Europe and northern Asia
	Rhipicephalinae (Metastriata)	*Dermacentor*	D. variabilis (American dog tick)	North America
			D. andersoni (Rocky Mountain wood tick)	North America
			D. reticulatus	Europe
	Rhipicephalinae (Metastriata)	*Rhipicephalus*	R. sanguineus (brown dog tick)	Worldwide
	Haemaphysalinae (Metastriata)	*Haemaphysalis*	H. leachi	Southern Africa
			H. bispinosa	Middle East, Africa, Asia
			H. longicornis	Middle East, Africa, Asia, Oceania
	Amblyomminae (Metastriata)	*Amblyomma*	A. americanum (lone star tick)	North America
			A. maculatum (Gulf coast tick)	North America
			A. variegatum (tropical bont tick)	Africa

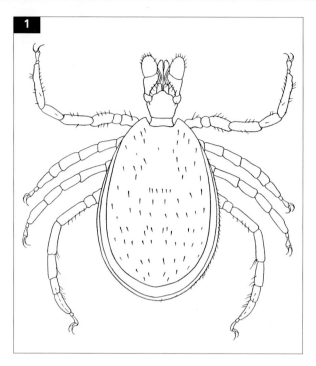

1 Adult male hard tick, *Ixodes ricinus*, in dorsal view. Ixodid ticks are relatively large, ranging between 2 and 20 mm in length. The body of the unfed tick is divided into only two sections: the anterior gnathosoma, which bears the mouthparts (the chelicerae, hypostome and palps), and a posterior idiosoma, which bears the legs. Ticks do not possess antennae and when eyes are present they are simple and are located dorsally at the sides of the scutum. (Reproduced from Savory TH (1935) *The Arachnida*. Edward Arnold & Co., London)

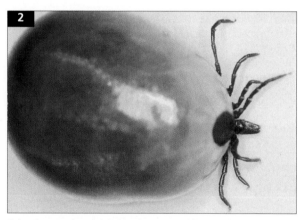

2 *Ixodes* species. Adult female removed from a dog.

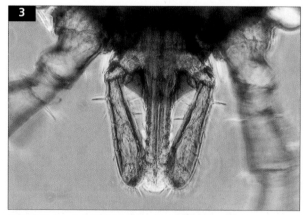

3 *Ixodes* species. Higher power magnification of the gnathosoma of an *Ixodes* species nymph removed from the coat of a dog.

domestic livestock. Its range is believed to be increasing with warmer wetter winters, and feeding on dogs and cats may occur over extended periods of the year. The hedgehog tick, *I. hexagonus*, is widely distributed throughout Europe in peri-urban environments, and in north-west Africa. In Europe, *I. hexagonus* may be the tick most commonly found on cats. *Dermacentor* species are also frequently encountered in North America and southern and central Europe. Dogs are the preferred hosts of adult *D. variabilis* (American dog tick) while larvae and nymphs feed largely on small rodents. Adults are most abundant from late spring to early summer but in some areas may persist until autumn.

Morphology

Ixodid ticks are relatively large (2–20 mm in length) (1–3). The mouthparts are composed of a pair of four-segmented palps (simple sensory organs), which aid host location. Between the palps lies a pair of heavily sclerotized, segmented appendages called chelicerae, housed in cheliceral sheaths. At the end of each chelicera are a number of tooth-like digits. The chelicerae are capable of moving back and forth and the tooth-like digits are used to cut and pierce the skin of the host animal during feeding. Below the chelicerae is the median hypostome, which emerges from the base of the palps (the basis capituli) and extends anteriorly and ventrally. The hypostome does not move but is armed with rows of backwardly directed, ventral teeth. The hypostome is thrust into the hole cut by the chelicerae and the teeth are used to attach the tick securely to its host. As the hypostome is inserted, the palps are spread flat onto the surface of the host's skin.

During feeding, hard ticks may remain attached to their host for several days. For ticks with long mouthparts, attachment by the chelicerae and hypostome is sufficient to anchor the tick in place. However, for ticks with short mouthparts, attachment is maintained during feeding by salivary secretions that harden around the mouthparts and effectively cement the tick in place.

Female ticks can increase in size substantially when they engorge during feeding. Some of the larger species of *Amblyomma* can increase from just under 10 mm to over 25 mm in length and increase from about 0.04 g to over 4 g in weight during feeding. The dorsal surface of male hard ticks is covered by a hardened protective shield (scutum); this is greatly reduced in females. As a result, males are not able to engorge to the same degree as females and may take more frequent smaller meals.

Life cycle

The life cycle of ixodid ticks involves four stages: egg, six-legged larva, eight-legged nymph and eight-legged adult (**4**). During passage through these stages the larvae, nymphs and adults take a number of blood meals. Tick parasitism probably evolved through close association with nest-dwelling (nidiculous) hosts until mechanisms developed that allowed them to remain permanently on their host or to locate and relocate hosts at intervals in the open environment.

Most, though not all, non-nidiculous hard ticks adopt a 'sit and wait' strategy rather than actively searching for hosts. To obtain a blood meal, they climb to the tips of vegetation, usually to a height appropriate for their host. This behaviour is described as 'questing'. Ticks identify a potential host via chemoreceptors on the tarsi of their first pair of legs, using cues such as carbon dioxide and other semiochemicals emitted by the host. Following contact, they transfer to the host and move over the skin surface to find their preferred attachment sites.

For most ixodid ticks, living in an environment where there is a relatively plentiful supply of host animals and in

4 The three-host feeding strategy of an ixodid tick. On finding a suitable host, usually a small mammal or bird, the larvae of ixodid ticks begin to feed. Blood feeding typically takes between four and six days. On completion of feeding, the larvae drop to the ground where they moult to become nymphs. After another interval, the nymphs begin to quest for a second host and, after feeding, drop to the ground and moult to become adults. Finally, after a further interval, adults begin to quest and females mate and engorge on their final host. After the final blood meal, adult females drop to the ground where they lay large batches of several thousand eggs over a period of days or weeks. Adult males may remain unattached on the host animal and attempt to mate with as many females as possible.

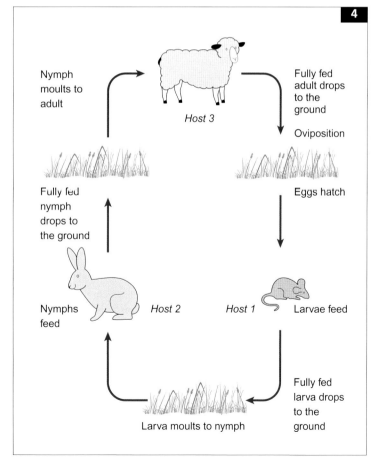

habitats where conditions are suitable for good survival during the off-host phase, a three-host life cycle has been adopted (4). For example, the deer tick *Ixodes scapularis* is a vector of the spirochaetes of *Borrelia burgdorferi* in North America. Larval *I. scapularis* become infected after feeding on small rodents, particularly the white-footed mouse. Bacteria are then transmitted from larval to nymphal and adult stages (trans-stadial transmission). The preferred host for adult ticks is the white-tailed deer. Therefore, Lyme borreliosis is generally confined to locations where the vector tick, the disease reservoir (the white-footed mouse) and the preferred host (the white-tailed deer) are abundant.

For the relatively small number of ixodid ticks (about 50 species) that inhabit areas where hosts are scarce and lengthy seasonal periods of unfavourable climate occur (e.g. *Rhipicephalus bursa* or *Dermacentor albipictus*), two- and one-host feeding strategies have evolved, respectively.

For many non-nidiculous ticks, the ancestral nest-dwelling habit is reflected in their selective environmental requirements, particularly for high relative humidity. For example, *I. ricinus* begins to quest when temperatures rise above a critical threshold of about 7°C (44.6°F) but requires a humidity above 80% to survive and feed. These environmental constraints restrict feeding activity to relatively short periods of the year during spring and autumn. Outside these periods, ticks remain quiescent, sheltering within the vegetation. Clearly, since tick densities and geographical and temporal activity ranges are strongly determined by microclimate, these may be greatly extended by climate change, particularly mild wet winters.

Vectorial potential

Almost all the ticks of importance as vectors of disease in cats and dogs are three-host species, and it is this movement between different types of vertebrate hosts, and the fact that they are not strictly host-specific in their feeding preferences, that make ticks such important disease vectors. Wild animals are particularly important as reservoirs of pathogens through a wild animal/tick/domestic animal cycle of contact (see Chapter 2). Several other factors contribute to the vectorial capacity of ticks. These include: secure attachment to their host; lengthy feeding periods allowing large numbers of pathogens to be ingested and transmitted; high rates of reproduction; and the transmission of pathogens between tick life cycle-stages (trans-stadial transmission) and between generations via the egg (transovarial transmission) (see Chapter 2). Infection of a host with tick-transmitted pathogens may be aided by salivary anticoagulants and other active compounds that modulate host cutaneous immunity and inflammation, while enhancing vasodilation in order to bring more blood to the feeding site (see Chapter 3). The salivary fluid is the principal avenue for disease transmission in the hard ticks.

FLEAS

Fleas (order Siphonaptera) are small, wingless, obligate, blood-feeding insects. The order is relatively small, with about 2,500 described species. On cats and dogs, *Ctenocephalides felis* and *Ctenocephalides canis* are the two species of major importance worldwide. However, in most geographical areas, even on dogs, *C. felis* predominates.

Morphology and life cycle

Adult fleas are highly modified for an ectoparasitic life and are structurally very different from most other insects (5). In contrast to lice or ticks, the flea body is laterally compressed. Adults are wingless and usually between 1 mm and 6 mm in length, with females being larger than males. The mouthparts are modified for piercing, with a salivary canal for injecting saliva into the wound and a food canal along which blood is drawn. Both sexes are blood feeders.

At 24°C (75.2°F) and 78% relative humidity (RH), and with a plentiful food supply, under most household conditions, *C. felis* will complete its developmental cycle

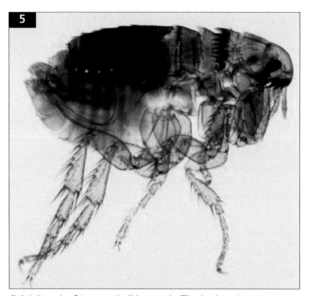

5 Adult male *Ctenocephalides canis*. The body colour may vary from light brown to black. The body is divided into head, thorax and abdomen, which are armed with spines that are directed backward. The head is high, narrow and cuneate. Eyes are absent in some species of nest flea but if present, they are usually simple and found on the head in front of the antennae. The shape of the abdomen may be used to distinguish the sexes. In female fleas, both ventral and dorsal surfaces are rounded. In the male flea the dorsal surface is relatively flatter and the ventral surface greatly curved.

in 3–5 weeks (**6**). However, under adverse conditions this can be extended to as long as 190 days. The eggs cannot withstand major variations in temperature and will not survive below 50% RH. At 70% RH and 35°C (95°F), 50% of *C. felis* eggs hatch within 1.5 days. At 70% RH and 15°C (59°F), it takes six days for 50% of eggs to hatch. The duration of the three larval stages is about one week at 24°C (75.2°F) and 75% RH, but in unfavourable conditions the larval cycle can take up to 200 days. Larvae will only survive at temperatures between 13°C (55.4°F) and 35°C (95°F) and mortality is high below 50% RH. The duration of the pupal stage is about 8–9 days at 24°C (75.2°F) and 78% RH.

When fully developed, adults emerge from the pupal cuticle but may remain within the cocoon for up to 12 months at low temperatures. Emergence may be extremely rapid under optimal conditions and is triggered by mechanical pressure, changes in light, vibrations, elevated carbon dioxide and heat. As adult fleas generally do not actively search for hosts and hosts may only return to the lair or bedding at infrequent intervals, the ability to remain within the cocoon for extended periods is essential. The air currents created by warm, mobile objects in close proximity induce adult cat fleas to jump. Once on their host, *C. felis* adults feed almost immediately and tend to become permanent residents. Within 36 hours of adult emergence, most females will have found hosts and mated. Egg laying begins 24–48 hours after the first blood meal.

Vectorial potential

Fleas feed by piercing the skin of the host and inserting the tip of the labrum-epipharynx to extract capillary blood. A female flea consumes an average of 14 microlitres of blood per day. Fleas are vectors of a range of viruses and bacteria and pathogen transmission is enhanced by their promiscuous feeding habits. Most species of flea are host-preferential rather than host-specific and will try to feed on any available animal. For example, *C. felis* has been found on over fifty different host species. Other factors that contribute to the potential of *C. felis* as a vector include transovarial transmission of some pathogens (*Rickettsia* species) and the transmission of pathogens such as *Bartonella henselae* through adult flea faeces (see Chapters 10 and 12).

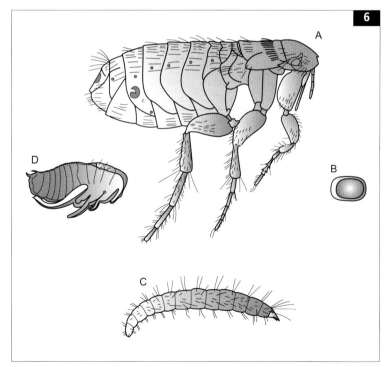

6 Life cycle of a typical flea. (A) Adult. Within 24–48 hours of the first blood meal, adult females begin to oviposit. The eggs may be deposited on the host but will fall to the ground within a few hours. Timing of oviposition may contribute to the concentration of flea eggs at the resting sites used by the host. In the laboratory, an adult female *C. felis* can produce an average of about 30 eggs per day over a life of about 50–100 days. However, on a cat or dog, the average life span is substantially less than this. (B) Egg. Flea eggs are about 0.5 mm in length, pearly white and oval. (C) Larva. Flea larvae are white and maggot-like with a distinct brownish head and they are covered with short hairs. Larvae grow in length from about 1.5 mm on hatching to 4–10 mm when fully grown. They have limited powers of movement (probably less than 20 cm before pupation) and are negatively phototactic and positively geotactic. In the domestic environment this behaviour often takes them to the base of carpets. Outdoors, they move into shaded areas under bushes, trees and leaves. Adult flea faeces are the primary food source for all three larval stages. (D) Pupa. When fully developed, the mature third-stage larva spins a thin, silk cocoon within which the larva pupates. Fragments of detritus, soil and dust adhere to the cocoon, giving it some degree of camouflage and protection from insecticides. (After Seguy E (1944) *Insectes Ectoparasites: Mallophages, Anopioures, Siphonapteres*. Lechevalier, Paris)

MOSQUITOES

The mosquitoes, family Culicidae, are a diverse family of true flies (Diptera), containing over 3,000 species. The family occurs worldwide from the Tropics to the Arctic and is divided into three subfamilies: Anophelinae, Culicinae and Toxorhynchitinae. There are more than 2,500 species of Culicinae, of which the main genera are *Aedes*, containing over 900 species, and *Culex*, with nearly 750 species.

Morphology and life cycle

Mosquitoes are small, slender flies, 2–10 mm in length (7). Anopheline and culicine mosquitoes can be readily differentiated on morphological and behavioural characteristics (8).

Mosquitoes lay their eggs on the surface of water on damp ground, usually at night. They often deposit more than 200 eggs per oviposition. The larvae of all species are aquatic and they occur in a wide variety of habitats such as the edge of permanent pools, puddles, flooded tree-holes or even temporary water-filled containers. Mosquito larvae require between three and 20 days to pass through four stadia. The final larval stage moults to become a pupa and this stage may last between one and seven days. Mating normally occurs within 24 hours of emergence and is completed in flight. Mosquitoes feed on nectar and plant juices, but females need a blood meal to develop their ovaries and must feed between each egg batch. Longevity is highly variable and species-specific, but on average, females live for 2–3 weeks, while the male lifespan is shorter.

Mosquitoes are nocturnal or crepuscular feeders, with a wide host range. Host location is achieved using a range of olfactory and visual cues, orientation to wind direction and body warmth. Mosquitoes typically require four days to digest a blood meal and produce eggs. Oviposition begins as soon as a suitable site is located. Adult mosquitoes are strong fliers, anopheline species in particular.

Vectorial potential

When mosquitoes feed, both the mandibles and the maxillae puncture the skin. Saliva passes down the salivary canal in the hypopharynx while blood passes up the food canal formed by the elongated labrum. Mosquitoes act as vectors for a range of viral, nematode and protozoan pathogens. Mosquito vectors can be relatively long lived and may overwinter, allowing pathogen survival from one season to another. When competent mosquitoes feed on the blood of a viraemic vertebrate host, virions are ingested with the blood meal and enter the midgut epithelial cells, within which they replicate. After spreading to the haemocoele, they then disperse to a variety of tissues, particularly the salivary glands, fat bodies, ovaries and nerves. Salivary transmission of the virus occurs when the infected mosquito next feeds on an appropriate host. In some mosquitoes, transovarial transmission of viruses also occurs. Mosquitoes are also vectors of the canine heartworm *Dirofilaria immitis* (see Chapter 5).

Different mosquito species have different blood feeding preferences; some will feed only on certain hosts while others are less discriminating and will feed on a variety of hosts depending on their relative abundance. *Culex quinquefasciatus*, for example, frequently feed on dogs but less frequently on cats. This host species preference might explain why dogs are more commonly infected with heartworm than cats.

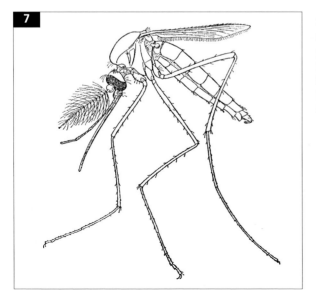

7 Adult male mosquito, *Aedes aegypti*. Adult mosquitoes have scales on the wing veins and margins and adult females possess an elongated proboscis, which is used in blood feeding. Male mosquitoes have plumose antennae, whereas those of females have fewer, shorter hairs. (Reproduced from Snodgrass RE (1935) *Principles of Insect Morphology*. McGraw Hill Book Company, New York)

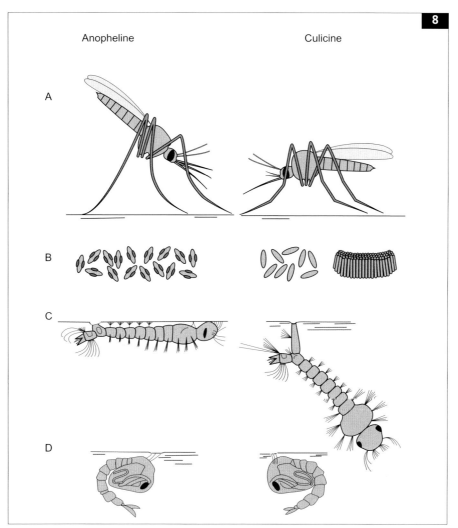

8 Key life cycle features distinguishing anopheline and culicine mosquitoes. (A) Adults. Living anopheline adults can readily be distinguished from culicines, such as *Aedes* and *Culex*, when resting on a flat surface. On landing, anopheline mosquitoes rest with the proboscis, head, thorax and abdomen in one straight line at an angle to the surface. The culicine adult rests with its body angled and its abdomen directed towards the surface. The palps of female anopheline mosquitoes are as long and straight as the proboscis, whereas in female culicine mosquitoes the palps are usually only about one-quarter of the length of the proboscis. The abdomen of *Anopheles* bears hairs but not scales. (B) Eggs. The eggs of anopheline mosquitoes possess characteristic lateral floats that maintain their orientation in the water and prevent them from sinking. Most species of *Aedes* lay their eggs on moist substrates, where they await adequate water to stimulate hatching. *Culex* form batches of eggs into a raft on the water surface. (C) Larvae. Anopheline larvae lie parallel to the water surface and breathe through a pair of spiracles at the posterior end of the abdomen. In contrast, culicine larvae hang suspended from the water surface by a prominent posterior breathing siphon, with spiracles at its tip. *Culex* and *Aedes* larvae feed by filtering out microorganisms from the water using mouth brushes. Anopheline larvae collect particles from the air-water interface. (D) Pupae. Mosquito pupae usually remain at the water surface but when disturbed they can be highly mobile. They do not feed during this phase and breathe by means of respiratory siphons. Adult mosquitoes emerge from the pupal case and crawl from the water to harden their cuticle and inflate their wings.

SANDFLIES

The Psychodidae is large family of true flies (Diptera) containing over 600 species. Within this family, the subfamily Phlebotominae includes biting species known as sandflies. They are widely distributed in the Tropics, Subtropics and around the Mediterranean. There are two genera of Phlebotominae of veterinary importance: in the Old World, *Phlebotomus*, and in the New World, *Lutzomyia*. Sandflies transmit the important zoonotic protozoal infection leishmaniosis in dogs and cats.

Morphology and life cycle

Phlebotomine sandflies are narrow bodied and up to five mm in length (**9**). They breed in humid, terrestrial habitats. Females lay 50–100 eggs per egg batch in small cracks or holes in damp ground, leaf litter and around the roots of forest trees. The larvae pass through four stadia before pupation and they feed on organic debris (faeces and decaying plant material). The life cycle is slow and takes at least 7–10 weeks, with many Palaearctic species having only two generations per year. Adult sandflies feed on nectar, sap, honeydew and fruit juices and live for 2–6 weeks. Only adult females are blood feeders. Adults often accumulate in refugia where the microclimate is suitable for breeding (e.g. rodent burrows and caves), with females blood feeding on the mammals in close vicinity. They have very limited powers of flight, moving in characteristic short hops, and have a range of perhaps only 100–200 metres.

Vectorial potential

When blood feeding, the toothed mandibles cut the skin while the maxillae hold the mouthparts in place in the wound. Blood is sucked from a subcutaneous pool and up a food canal formed by the labium above and the hypopharynx below. The salivary duct is formed by the under side of the hypopharynx. Blood feeding is limited to areas of exposed, less densely haired areas of skin, such as the ears, eyelids, nose, feet and tail. The feeding activity of most species occurs during dusk or even darkness, although some will bite during daylight. Most sandflies have a broad host range.

Sandflies are important as vectors of canine and feline leishmaniosis (see Chapter 8). *Leishmania* amastigotes are ingested with a blood meal when sandflies feed on an infected host, and they develop extracellularly in the mid- and hindgut. After three days, they transform into promasigotes and migrate into the foregut, where multiplication occurs. Infective promastigotes are regurgitated from the mouthparts, foregut and midgut into the dermis of a new host during feeding. This process is assisted by blockage of the foregut caused by congregated parasites, which prevents the fly from feeding effectively, thus ensuring repeated feeding attempts on multiple hosts. Infection is assisted by the presence of vasodilatory enzymes and immunomodulatory chemicals in the fly saliva (see Chapter 3).

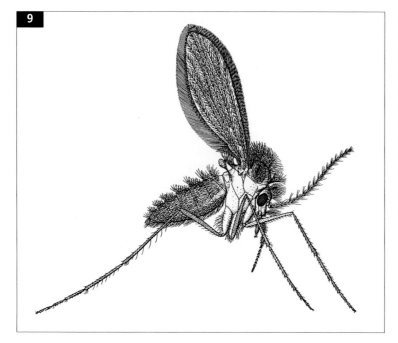

9

9 Adult female sandfly, *Phlebotomus papatasi*. Phlebotomines are densely hairy in appearance, with large black eyes and long legs. The wings are narrow, long, hairy and held erect over the thorax when at rest. The antennae are long, 16-segmented, filamentous and covered in fine setae. The thorax is strongly humped. The larvae are elongate, legless and up to five mm in length, with a distinct head carrying eyespots and toothed mandibles. (Reproduced from Smart JA (1943) *Handbook for the Identification of Insects of Medical Importance.* British Museum (Natural History), London)

TABANID AND MUSCID FLIES

The Tabanidae and Muscidae are large and important families of true flies (Diptera). Most species of veterinary importance belong to one of three genera: *Tabanus* (horse flies, greenheads), *Chrysops* (deer flies) and *Haematopota* (clegs). The family Muscidae contains several species (*Musca domestica*, *M. sorbens*, *M. autumnalis* and *M. vetustissima*) that may be important mechanical vectors of disease and some that are also blood feeding (*Haematobia irritans*). The family also includes the stable fly *Stomoxys calcitrans*, which is of importance as a biting fly of many mammalian hosts, including dogs. The stable fly is now found worldwide, after being introduced into North America from Europe during the 1700s. *Stomoxys niger* and *S. sitiens* may replace *S. calcitrans* as important blood feeding pests in Afrotropical and Oriental regions.

Morphology and life cycles

All the Tabanidae are large robust flies (**10**). The adults are strong fliers and are usually diurnal. Both sexes feed on nectar and, in most species, females are also blood feeders on a wide range of hosts. The tabanids are painful and persistent biters.

Tabanid eggs are laid in large masses and hatch after 4–7 days. The first-stage larvae move to mud or wet soil and quickly moult. The larvae of *Chrysops* may feed on decaying vegetable debris, while those of *Haematopota* and *Tabanus* are carnivorous; therefore, the latter species are often found at relatively low population densities. Most larvae require periods of several months to several years to complete development, during which time they pass through six and 13 stadia. Pupation takes place close to, or within, dryer soil and requires 2–3 weeks. The life cycle length varies from 10–42 weeks. Most temperate species have only a single generation per year and adults live for 2–4 weeks.

Both sexes of *S. calcitrans* are persistent and strong fliers and are active by day. Female adults are 5–7 mm in length. The body is usually grey, with seven circular black spots on its abdomen and four dark longitudinal stripes on its thorax. Stable flies have piercing and sucking mouthparts, with short maxillary palps, and both sexes are blood feeders. After multiple blood meals, adult females lay eggs in wet straw, garden debris, old stable bedding or manure. Eggs hatch in 5–10 days, depending on temperature. The cream-coloured, saprophagous larvae pass through three stadia and then pupariate. The life cycle length varies from 3–7 weeks, depending on temperature.

Vectorial potential

Tabanid mouthparts are short and strong for slashing, rasping and sponging. They are important mechanical vectors of several viral, bacterial, protozoan and nematode pathogens. When a female tabanid feeds, saliva containing an anticoagulant is pumped into the wound, before blood is sucked up into the food canal. When feeding ceases, the labia of the mouthparts trap a small quantity of blood. Pathogens in this blood may be protected for an hour or more and successfully transmitted to a new host at the next meal. Mechanical transmission is made more likely by the painful nature of tabanid bites. Biting flies are more likely to be dislodged by the host before blood feeding is complete and they will attempt to feed again rapidly, increasing the chance of live pathogen transmission.

Stable flies also inflict frequent, painful bites and remain on their hosts only when feeding. They will occasionally follow potential hosts for considerable distances and will follow them indoors. Stable flies are known mechanically to transmit a number of viral pathogens and are also suspected of transmitting bacteria, protozoa and nematodes.

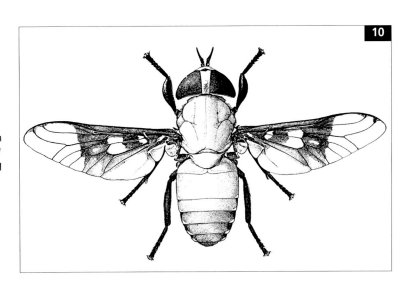

10 A tabanid, *Tabanus latipes*. The body is generally dark in colour, although this can be variable, ranging from dull brown to black or grey. Some species may even be brilliant yellow, green or metallic blue. However, the body also usually carries a pattern of stripes or pale patches and the thorax and abdomen are covered with fine hairs. (Reproduced from Castellani A and Chalmers AJ (1919) *Manual of Tropical Medicine*. 3rd edn. Baillière, Tindall and Cox, London)

TRUE BUGS

The order Hemiptera, known as the true bugs, includes roughly 90,000 insect species. They all have piercing and sucking mouthparts and two pairs of wings. Most of the species feed only on plant juices. However, species of the family Ruduviidae are of medical and veterinary significance as all species can transmit the protozoan *Trypanosoma cruzi*, the causative agent of Chagas' disease (see Chapter 13).

Morphology and life cycle

Adult bugs are secretive, hiding in cracks and crevices in buildings and natural habitats. Eggs are laid in groups or loosely on a substrate and they hatch within 10–30 days. There are usually five stadia before the insects reach maturity, the nymphs being similar in appearance to adults but not possessing wings and being capable of moulting to the next stage after only one blood meal (**11**). Depending on temperature, the life cycle may be completed in 3–6 months but usually requires 1–2 years.

Vectorial potential

Feeding is initiated by chemical and physical cues. Carbon dioxide causes increased activity and heat will stimulate probing. When probing is initiated, the rostrum is swung forward and the mandibular stylets are used to cut through the skin and then anchor the mouthparts. The maxillary stylets probe for a blood vessel and saliva containing an anticoagulant passes down the salivary canal while blood is pumped up the food canal. Feeding may take between three and 30 minutes. After engorging, the rostrum is removed from the host and the bug defecates, after which it crawls away to find shelter. If the bug feeds on a host infected with *Trypanosoma cruzi*, amastigotes or trypomastigotes may be ingested. In the vector the parasite reproduces asexually and metacyclic trypomastigotes develop in its hindgut. The next time the bug feeds, metacyclic trypomastigotes are voided in its faeces and are rubbed or scratched into the bite wound or mucous membranes of the eye, nose or mouth. The interval between feeding and defecation is critical in determining the effectiveness of disease transmission.

CONTROL

When dealing with arthropod-transmitted infections, prevention of arthropod attack is desirable as even low levels of biting may be sufficient to result in transmission. However, chemicals used for this purpose, particularly when applied to the environment, may be expensive and result in effects on non-target organisms and selection for resistance. Therefore, the choice of product requires detailed consideration of the vector species in question, its behaviour and biology, the mechanism and kinetics of transmission of infection and the level of infectious challenge.

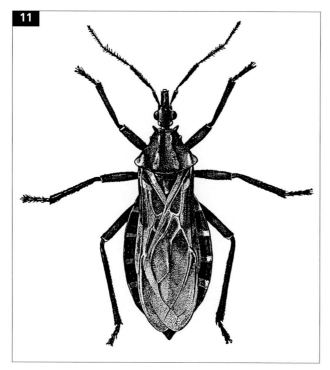

11 A cone-nosed bug, *Triatoma megistus*, in dorsal view. Triatomine bugs are generally between 20 and 30 mm in length. Most species are dark in colour but are often characteristically marked along the abdomen, pronotum or at the base of the wings with contrasting splashes of yellow, orange or red. They possess an elongated head with large eyes and four-segmented antennae. The segmented rostrum is formed by the labium, which encloses the stylet-like mouthparts, composed by the modified maxillae and mandibles used to pierce the skin of the host. When the bug is not feeding the rostrum is folded back under the head. An adult bug can take up to three times its own weight in blood. They feed roughly every 5–10 days, although they can survive prolonged periods without blood. (Reproduced from Castellan, A and Chalmers AJ (1919) *Manual of Tropical Medicine*. 3rd edn. Baillière, Tindall and Cox, London)

Over the past ten years, the problems associated with direct treatment of the environment have encouraged increased development of products for topical or systemic administration to small companion animals. These include a number of newer generation insecticidal and acaricidal chemicals such as fipronil, imidacloprid, nitenpyram and selemectin, as well as reformulations of existing compounds such as amitraz and the pyrethroids permethrin and deltamethrin. Many of the newer products are highly arthropod specific, resulting in increased mammalian safety. In addition, they have prolonged residual activity, thus decreasing the frequency of administration. Products combining ectoparasiticides with insect development inhibitors such as methoprene and lufenuron are now available for on-animal use. Formulations for on-animal use are varied, although many of the newer drugs are 'spot-on' preparations. Others include sprays, dips, collars, shampoos, foams and powders, as well as oral preparations. Environmental treatments suitable for domestic premises include traditional insecticides (organophosphates, carbamates, pyrethrins) either alone or in combination with insect growth regulators, and biological control using nematodes.

Although there are several management strategies available for control of arthropods on dogs and cats, control of arthropod vectors in wildlife reservoirs still remains a major challenge.

Tick control

Animals should be inspected for ticks daily, particularly during the spring and summer. On cats and dogs, the majority of adult ticks attach to the front of the body, particularly the ears, face, neck and interdigital areas. However, there may be variation between tick species in this respect. Larvae and nymphs may also be found along the dorsum. Attached ticks should be removed from cats and dogs using purpose-designed tick-removing tools. Jerking, twisting or crushing ticks during removal should be avoided. They should not be handled without gloves and, once removed, should be disposed of carefully.

Where practicable, contact between pets and known areas of high tick density should be limited at times of year when tick activity is known to be high. There are several acaricides developed for use on dogs and cats (*Table 3*, overleaf), and those that kill or repel ticks before or soon after they attach are particularly valuable. Environmental treatment with organophosphates or pyrethroids in domestic premises may be useful under some circumstances. However, since off-host life cycle stages are often in highly inaccessible locations, environmental treatment is usually of only limited efficacy.

Flea control

For optimal control of flea-transmitted infections, the adults already infesting dogs and cats should be killed immediately and reinfestation from the environment prevented. A wide range of products is available (*Table 3*). Many of the new chemicals with excellent long-acting flea adulticidal activity also have contact ovicidal and/or larvicidal activity. In addition, combination with insect growth regulators (chitin synthesis inhibitors, juvenile hormone analogues) applied directly to the animal not only increases ovicidal and/or larvicidal activity but also delivers it effectively to the sleeping areas most likely to be infested, without unnecessarily contaminating the environment. Insect growth regulators do not kill adult fleas and are not suitable by themselves for controlling flea-transmitted diseases, unless used in a completely closed environment. Frequent vacuuming can help to reduce environmental infestation and pet bedding should be washed at high temperatures.

Fly control

The most effective method to prevent fly bites and transmission of infection is to ensure that pets avoid areas of high fly density and are kept indoors when fly activity is highest. Flies spend a limited time on their hosts and are difficult to control using insecticides unless these have rapid killing or repellent activity. Permethrin and deltamethrin are the only insecticides with sufficient repellent activity and rapidity of action to make them suitable for the control of sandfly biting in dogs (*Table 3*). Neither insecticide is suitable for cats.

The environmental use of residual insecticides is difficult for insects that do not have readily identified breeding or resting sites. Tabanid and many muscid larvae are generally inaccessible to insecticides. Most adult insect vectors are relatively strong fliers and can move several miles from where they developed as larvae. Hence, successful control of larvae in one site may not result in significant reductions in adult fly numbers, biting activity or disease transmission. In some countries, public control agencies are responsible for controlling mosquito and other vector numbers. In areas where mosquito and other fly populations are problematic, the domestic environment may be protected by fine mesh window and door screens, draining standing water or treating it with chemical insecticides or the microbial insecticide produced by *Bacillus thuringiensis* subspecies *israelensis*. The use of any insecticide product should be combined with good sanitation practices that reduce breeding sites.

Triatomine control

Domestic bugs can be controlled by spraying dwellings with formulations of pyrethroid insecticide. This is often enough to eliminate existing populations of the bugs within a house, although reintroductions are possible.

Table 3 Insecticides, acaricides and insect growth regulators used in the control of arthropod infestations of dogs and cats.

Active ingredient	Product	Action on arthropod vectors	Application
Fipronil (phenylpyrazole)	Frontline, Frontline Plus, Frontline Combo (Merial)	Neurotoxin; inhibits GABA-mediated receptors in the arthropod CNS; flea adulticide, acaricide. When formulated with methoprene, flea larvicide	Topical spot-on, spray
Imidocloprid (chloronicotinyl, pyridylmethylamine)	Advantage, Advantix for dogs (Bayer)	Neurotoxin; inhibits nicotinergic-mediated receptors. Flea adulticide. When formulated with permethrin will kill and repel ticks and flies in dogs	Topical spot-on
Selamectin (macrocyclic-lactone)	Stronghold, Revolution (Pfizer)	Neurotoxin; binds to glutamate-gated chloride channels in the arthropod CNS; flea adulticide and larvicide. Some acaricidal activity	Topical spot-on
Amitraz (triazapentadiene)	Mitaban (Upjohn), Aludex (Intervet), Preventic (Allerderm/Virbac) and various generic brands	Neurotoxin; action not fully understood; insecticide and acaricide	Collar or topical pour-on
Nitenpyram (neonicotinoid, pyridylmethylamine)	Capstar (Novartis)	Neurotoxin; binds and inhibits insect-specific nicotinic acetylcholine receptors; rapid acting flea adulticide	Oral
Organophosphates (e.g. malathion, ronnel, chlorpyrifos, fenthion, dichlorvos, cythioate, diazanon) propetamphos, phosmet	Various	Neurotoxins; cholinesterase inhibitors; general adulticides	Topical or systemic formulations, plus environmental preparations
Carbamates (e.g. carbaryl, propoxur, bendiocarb)	Various	Neurotoxins; cholinesterase inhibitors; general adulticides	Topical or environmental preparations
Pyrethroids (e.g. permethrin, deltamethrin, others)	Various	Neurotoxins; synthetic insecticides derived from pyrethrins; interfere with sodium activation gate of the nerve cells; tick, flea, fly adulticide and repellent. Do not use in cats	Topical or environmental preparations
Lufenuron (benzoyl phenylurea)	Program (Novartis)	Chitin synthesis inhibitor. Flea ovicide and some larvicidal activity	Oral or depot injection
Cyromazine	Staykil (Novartis)	Insect growth inhibitor. Flea larvicide	Environmental preparation
Methoprene, pyriproxifen	Various	Juvenile hormone and juvenile hormone analogues. Flea larvicide	Environmental preparations, collars, spot-ons
Natural botanical products (eucalyptus oil, pennyroyal oil, tea tree oil, citrus oil and D-limonene, rotenone)	Various	Insecticidal or insect repellent properties. However, the precise efficacy unknown. Neurotoxity after ingestion at high concentrations. Do not use in cats	Topical

The role of wildlife and wildlife reservoirs in the maintenance of arthropod-borne infections

Kevin Bown and Malcolm Bennett

INTRODUCTION

As interest in emerging microparasitic infections of human and domestic animals such as *Borrelia burgdorferi*, *Anaplasma phagocytophilum* and *Bartonella* species has grown in recent decades, the key role of wildlife in their maintenance has led to increased interest in the ecology of these agents in their natural hosts. While much is still unknown, it is becoming apparent that complex interactions between hosts, vectors and microparasites (bacteria, viruses and protozoa) have evolved to enable the continued existence of such agents in natural systems. This chapter will highlight a number of wildlife species important in the maintenance of arthropod-borne infections of dogs and cats, and some of the key ecological adaptations involved.

THE IMPORTANCE OF WILDLIFE IN THE MAINTENANCE OF ARTHROPOD-BORNE INFECTIONS

The concept of reservoir hosts

Wild animals have been implicated in the epidemiology of many arthropod-borne infections and, as more research into emerging diseases takes place, more wildlife reservoirs will be identified. Several of the infections discussed in detail elsewhere in this book are maintained in wildlife hosts, and infection and disease in humans and domesticated animals occurs only 'accidentally' as a result of being bitten by a vector. These accidental hosts play little role in maintaining the microparasite. Those species deemed essential for maintaining the infection within its natural ecological system are termed reservoir hosts. Such hosts must be susceptible to infection and allow the microparasite to reach the stage of development required for it to be transmitted. Infection can persist within populations of reservoir hosts in the absence of host species other than arthropod vectors, and infection in accidental host species usually results from contact, either directly or indirectly (i.e. via an arthropod vector), with a reservoir host. For example, dogs and cats can become infected with *Borrelia burgdorferi* if fed on by an infected tick that has, in turn, fed on an infected vole or mouse during an earlier developmental stage, but dogs and cats play no significant role in the overall epidemiology of the infection. In other cases, dogs and cats themselves may be reservoir hosts for an infection. For example, both wild and domestic species of cat appear to be the sole reservoir host for *Bartonella henselae* and *B. clarridgeiae*, while dogs appear to fill this role for *B. vinsonii* subspecies *berkhoffii*.

For many of the infections described in later chapters there is more than one reservoir species involved in maintaining the microparasite in nature, and as recognition of the potential role of wildlife increases, so more and more species are being implicated in the maintenance of vector-borne infections. For example *Anaplasma phagocytophilum* (previously *Ehrlichia phagocytophila*, *Cytocoetes phagocytophila*), the agent responsible for granulocytic ehrlichiosis in dogs and cats, has long been associated in Europe with disease in sheep and other ruminants, which were widely regarded as the principal reservoir hosts. However, within the past few years, small rodents have also been identified as reservoir hosts. The role rodents play in the epidemiology of disease in humans and domesticated animals remains unclear, not least as there is debate about whether all strains of *A. phagocytophilum* are identical, or whether each has its own host range and ecology and, consequently, is of different pathogenicity to accidental hosts such as dogs, cats and man.

Infection in reservoir and accidental hosts

A difference often commented on between the behaviour of arthropod-borne parasites in reservoir hosts and accidental hosts is in the pathogenesis of the infection and resultant disease. Many reservoir hosts show few clinical signs of infection. For example, there is little evidence of clinical disease in rodents with bartonellosis, babesiosis or granulocytic ehrlichiosis. This is not, however, a hard-and-fast rule, as some apparent reservoir hosts can become clinically diseased. For example, white-footed mice (*Peromyscus leucopus*) may exhibit neurological signs of infection with *Borrelia burgdorferi* despite being an important reservoir host for this bacterium. Furthermore, 'disease' can be difficult to detect in wildlife unless it causes high mortality or obvious lesions such as effects on fecundity, susceptibility to predation, ability to defend a territory or forage for food, or growth and maturation rates. Such parameters are difficult to study in wild populations, and data on such aspects of wildlife infections are scarce. However, while the selection pressures on hosts and parasites may often lead to the co-evolution of traits resulting in relatively subtle disease, no such selection occurs during infection of accidental hosts. Thus, although some accidental host species can have inapparent infections (in which case they will probably not be noticed), in others the same agent, expressing genes that have evolved for survival in reservoir hosts, may cause obvious disease. If these diseased, accidental hosts happen to be domesticated animals or human beings, then the causative agent will be much studied as a 'pathogen' even though the occurrence of disease in such hosts might be considered accidental.

The co-evolution of reservoir hosts and agents can lead to diverse ecological and pathogenic properties among apparently closely related agents. For example, while it is often thought that *Borrelia burgdorferi* (see Chapter 9) has a broad range of reservoir host species that includes rodents, lagomorphs, insectivores, birds and sheep, there is strong evidence for ecologically important relationships between a particular host species and the species of *Borrelia* for which it acts as reservoir. *B. afzelii*, for example, is mainly associated with rodents and *B. garinii* with birds. Recent studies suggest that the host ranges of these different species of *Borrelia* are determined by differences in their sensitivity to host complement. While *B. afzelii* is resistant to rodent complement and can thus survive and be acquired by a feeding tick such as *Ixodes ricinus*, it is sensitive to the complement of hosts such as birds. As such, a tick infected with *B. afzelii* by feeding on a rodent in one instar may lose that infection if it feeds on a bird during the next instar. These slight differences in phenotype, which enable closely related agents to each exploit their own ecological niches, can lead to differences in behaviour and, therefore, pathogenicity in accidental hosts. Within the species that make up the *Borrelia burgdorferi* complex, only some appear to be associated with specific clinical syndromes in dogs, cats and humans.

For example, Lyme arthritis is associated with *B. burgdorferi sensu stricto* infection, neuroborreliosis with *B. garinii* and *B. afzelii* is associated with acrodermatitis chronica atophicans (ACA). The pathogenic status of other *Borrelia* species such as *B. valaisiana* and *B. japonica* is currently uncertain (see Chapter 9).

Co-infection

It should be noted that wildlife species can also be important reservoir hosts for many different microparasites, and thus vectors feeding on them can acquire multiple infections and consequently transmit these to accidental hosts such as humans and companion animals. Wild rodents in the USA may be concurrently infected with *Borrelia burgdorferi*, *Babesia microti*, *Anaplasma phagocytophilum* and various *Bartonella* species, and similar findings have been reported in Europe. Whether there is any interaction between these microparasites is unclear but it would appear unlikely that a mixed infection could be any less pathogenic than a single one. In addition, in rodent communities, different rodent species may differ in their role as hosts to the various microparasites. For example, bank voles (*Clethrionomys glareolus* [12]) and wood mice (*Apodemus sylvaticus* [13]) in the UK are both reservoirs for the same community of *Bartonella* species at relatively high prevalences (up to 70%), but bank voles are significantly more likely to be infected with *A. phagocytophilum* than are wood mice, and each rodent species is infected with its own specific trypanosome. The mechanisms by which these differences occur are unclear but if hosts living in close proximity and exposed to similar microparasites differ in their response to such infections, it seems obvious that such microparasites may invoke vastly different responses in accidental hosts.

Hosts not regarded as being reservoirs for an infection can still be vitally important in the epidemiology of that infection. The possible 'sterilizing' effect on ticks infected with certain *Borrelia* species when they feed on some hosts has been mentioned already, and this can obviously reduce transmission of the parasite amongst a community of tick hosts. In contrast, many deer species appear to be poor hosts for *Borrelia burgdorferi* spirochaetes, as their complement has borreliacidal activity and transmission to and from ticks feeding on deer does not occur. Yet deer can still be a vital component of the epidemiology of borreliosis as they feed large numbers of adult ticks and thus contribute to the size of subsequent tick populations, the earlier instars of which feed on infected and infectious hosts such as mice (see *Box* right).

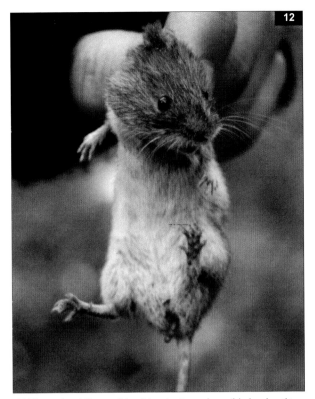

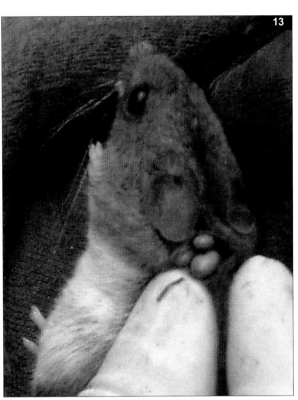

12 Throughout the world, wild rodents such as this bank vole (*Clethrionomys glareolus*) are important reservoir hosts for a multitude of vector-borne infections. This species alone is a reservoir for *Borrelia burgdorferi*, *Anaplasma phagocytophilum*, *Babesia microti*, various *Bartonella* species and tick-borne encephalitis virus.

13 Wood mouse (*Apodemus sylvaticus*) infested with adult *Ixodes trianguliceps* ticks.

The complex ecology of Lyme disease

A possible network of events has been described for Lyme disease in the eastern USA that illustrates the potential complexity of interactions that drive the dynamics of infections in wildlife, and can lead to outbreaks of disease in other hosts. The main host of *Borrelia burgdorferi sensu stricto* in the area is the white-footed mouse *Peromyscus leucopus*. Mouse population dynamics depend on the amount of food available, in particular acorn crop sizes in the large oak woodlands. A particularly large acorn yield (which itself depends on a number of environmental factors) leads to greater survival and fecundity of mice, with a consequent population explosion the following year. The ready availability of acorns also attracts deer to the same areas, and the deer harbour large numbers of adult ticks. These ticks lay their eggs, which hatch into larvae the following year – just in time to feed on the now greatly expanded mouse population. All of these factors combine to produce an explosion of *Borrelia*-infected nymphs and larvae and consequent outbreaks of Lyme disease in humans.

It has even been suggested that the emergence of human Lyme disease in the eastern USA might be a delayed consequence of the extinction of the passenger pigeon (*Ectopistes migratorius*) a century ago. Flocks of passenger pigeons are known to have migrated annually to areas with large crops of acorns, and there is some contemporary evidence that this effectively suppressed mouse populations and deer immigration. This in turn may have reduced the risk of Lyme disease to accidental hosts such as humans.

HOW ARE ARTHROPOD-BORNE INFECTIONS MAINTAINED BY WILDLIFE?

Basic epidemiology of infectious diseases

For any parasitic infection to persist it is essential that, on average, each infection results in at least one additional infection of another individual host. The number of new (or 'secondary') infections occurring as a result of each original (or 'primary') infection is termed the basic reproductive rate (R_0). Thus, in mathematical terms, for a microparasite to be maintained in a population, R_0 must be >1. If R_0 falls below one, then, over time, that microparasite will disappear from the population. Infection of incidental hosts such as cats and dogs may not lead to infection of another individual, due to physiological or ecological differences between themselves and reservoir hosts or as a result of veterinary treatment. Consequently, many accidental hosts are 'dead-end' hosts.

Mechanisms of persistence in wildlife populations

There are a number of obstacles to R_0 remaining greater than one. Passage of an infection from one host to another depends on a variety of factors. First, an infected host must encounter a competent vector, which must subsequently find and feed upon another suitable host, and thus the distribution and behaviour of vectors are crucial to understanding infection dynamics.

Distribution of vectors in the environment

The distribution of parasites in nature is not usually random but is aggregated (clumped) within the host population. This is generally true for all macroparasites, including nematodes, cestodes, insects and arachnids. This aggregation of parasites within a host population results in a situation where many of the individuals will be free from parasites, while a small proportion of individuals will be heavily parasitized. In fact, many host–parasite relationships have been shown to conform to the '20/80 rule', whereby 20% of the host population are burdened with 80% of the parasites. Two independent studies of the relationship between *I. ricinus* and rodent hosts reported that 20% of the rodents were infested with approximately 80% of the tick larvae and the majority of nymphs. Such an aggregated distribution has been shown essential for the maintenance of tick-borne encephalitis virus (TBEV) by enabling co-feeding transmission (see *Box* below) and by increasing R_0 by three or four.

There are a number of causes for aggregation of ticks in host populations, one of which is the manner in which female ticks lay eggs. Female ixodid ticks such as *I. ricinus* and *I. scapularis* lay a single, large egg mass after processing their final blood meal. Such egg masses can comprise several thousand eggs. If eggs from such masses hatch successfully, then within a relatively small area, several thousand questing larvae can be found. Any host in the area is thus likely to acquire a large number of larvae, while those hosts travelling in areas where egg masses are absent are unlikely to come into contact with larvae at all.

The foraging behaviour of ticks is another potential mechanism leading to their aggregation on hosts. Ticks use a number of cues to locate hosts including CO_2, NH_3, pheromones and body temperature. In cases where pheromones released by feeding females attract adult males to a host, it is obvious that this can result in aggregation of numbers of ticks on a host.

In addition to vector biology, there are several host-related factors that can influence parasite distribution within a population. One of the most important of these is host gender. Males of many species carry a higher parasite burden than females, one reason being that they have a larger territory. For example, male field voles (*Microtus agrestis*) have home ranges about twice the size as those of females. As a result, the chance of encountering parasites in the environment is much greater.

Co-feeding transmission between ticks

Within the past decade or so, the traditional view that arthropods could only acquire infections by feeding on hosts that were parasitaemic, or through transovarial transmission, has been shown to be incorrect. Co-feeding enables microparasite transmission between ticks in the absence of a host parasitaemia. This phenomenon, first reported for Thogoto virus, has since been demonstrated to be an important route of transmission for *Borrelia burgdorferi*, TBE group flaviviruses and possibly *Anaplasma phagocytophilum*. Co-feeding transmission increases the chances of transmission of microparasites such as TBEV, where the infected hosts are only infective to ticks for a few days or where parasitaemia never reaches infective levels. As ticks typically feed for between four days and two weeks, the period over which naïve ticks can acquire infection by feeding alongside infected ticks is greatly extended. Indeed, non-viraemic co-feeding transmission of TBEV may be essential for its persistence, and this is further aided by the high number of ticks found on individual hosts.

As well as increasing the period over which transmission can occur, co-feeding transmission also enables ticks to acquire infection while feeding on hosts that are immune to the microparasite infection. When rodents are challenged with TBEV they produce an immune response that clears the viraemia and protects them against further challenge. However, despite this apparent immunity, transmission can still occur between infected and naïve ticks via dendritic cells that take up the virus and then migrate to the feeding sites of other ticks. This enables immune wild rodents to continue to act as vectors of TBEV between ticks feeding on them.

Another possible way in which gender differences can affect parasite distribution is through the immuno-modulatory effects of sex hormones and consequent ability of the host to eliminate parasites. Experimental studies performed with male sand lizards (*Lacerta agilis*) implanted with testosterone showed that implanted males acquire heavier tick burdens than untreated males. This was postulated to be due to the immunosuppressive effects of testosterone. A further example can be found in bank voles. Bank voles are frequently exposed to ticks and they can develop a density-dependent immunity that results in both reduced attachment of ticks and significantly reduced feeding success of those ticks that attach successfully. However, testosterone can impair this acquired immunity in male bank voles. In addition, *Babesia microti* infections in bank voles given testosterone implants produce a more severe parasitaemia of longer duration than those in control animals. It is therefore apparent that certain groups within a host population, such as reproductively active males, may be of greater significance in the perpetuation of arthropod-borne infections than others.

The importance to microparasite transmission of cohorts determined by age and gender within a population is demonstrated by the following example. In a study of adult yellow-necked mice (*Apodemus flavicollis*), although only 26% of the individuals captured were males, they made up a significantly greater proportion of the population involved in transmission of TBEV. Therefore, in terms of disease control, targeting this group would be much more efficient than targeting the population as a whole.

In addition to determining the spatial distribution of vectors, host factors can sometimes determine their temporal distribution. An example is the intricate relationship that exists between *Spilopsyllus cuniculi* fleas and rabbits. Hormones released by female rabbits in late pregnancy are essential for the maturation of *Spilopsyllus* flea eggs, thus ensuring that emergence of the next generation of adult fleas coincides with the presence of newborn rabbits. In addition, growth hormone produced by newborn rabbits stimulates increased flea mating and feeding, thus maximizing productivity. Once the production of growth hormone declines, the fleas return to the mother and their reproduction halts.

An example of hosts determining both the spatial and temporal distribution of vectors has already been mentioned. Deer in North America, attracted to areas where the acorn crop is high, bring with them the adult ticks that will produce the larvae to feed on the following year's population of mice.

Environmental factors such as climate can also have a dramatic effect on parasite development and survival. For example, the distribution of TBEV can be predicted using satellite-derived data on environmental conditions. In rodents, which are generally regarded as the most important mammalian host for TBEV, detectable viraemia is rare and, when it does occur, is very short-lived. As a result, the transmission of TBEV relies heavily upon infected nymphs feeding in synchrony with naïve larval ticks to enable non-systemic co-feeding transmission (see *Box*, p. 26) to occur. This happens where summers are warm enough to allow rapid development of eggs, but also where autumns cool down quickly enough to force emerging larvae to overwinter without feeding. This results in both nymphs and larvae starting to quest at the same time the following spring.

Vector competence and microparasite acquisition

Once a vector has acquired infection, it must then feed on another competent host for the infection to perpetuate. Vector competence for some infections is less restricted than for others. Much depends on whether the mode of transmission is merely mechanical, where the vector acts as little more than a hypodermic needle, or biological, where the microparasite interacts in a more fundamental way (e.g. by replicating in the vector). Infections such as myxomatosis in rabbits persist as a result of mechanical transmission (see *Box*, p. 28) (**14**). In Australia and much

14 Rabbit showing clinical signs associated with myxomatosis. Infection in reservoir hosts is usually thought to be asymptomatic, but this is an obvious exception and an interesting study in the co-evolution of host and pathogen.

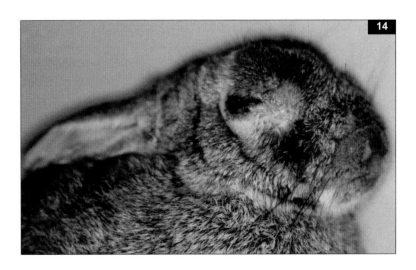

Myxomatosis – a disease in a reservoir host?

Rabbit myxomatosis illustrates an aspect of the relationship between host, agent and vector that is often misunderstood – that of the role sometimes played by disease. It is a common misconception that endemic infectious agents and their hosts will always co-evolve such that disease no longer occurs. Myxoma virus is endemic in rabbits of the genus *Sylvilagus* in southern USA and Central and South America, and in these hosts, with which it is assumed to have co-evolved over thousands of years, it causes little disease. Although such low pathogenicity in natural reservoir hosts is often the case, it is by no means a foregone conclusion. In susceptible European rabbits (*Oryctolagus cuniculus*), myxomatosis is a severe disease that often ends in the death of the host, and the co-evolution of myxoma virus and European rabbits, albeit over only half a century, provides an interesting model for study. When first introduced into rabbit populations in both Europe and Australia, there was certainly no selection against highly pathogenic strains of virus – in fact quite the opposite. Immediately after introduction, highly virulent strains of virus were selectively advantaged. Increased virulence was associated with a greater area of infected skin on which fleas and mosquitoes could feed and higher densities of virus in that tissue (and therefore on the vectors' mouthparts). Both factors combined to increase transmission. The virus strains with the highest R_0 were those with the highest virulence and pathogenicity – and the result for rabbit populations was catastrophic. However, as the number of susceptible rabbits plunged, acquired immunity and the selection of innately more resistant lines of rabbits reduced the population susceptible to infection and, therefore, the frequency of contact between infectious and susceptible hosts. At this stage, viral strains causing longer periods of infection had a selective advantage over more pathogenic strains, as they had a greater chance of being transmitted before the host died. Although this may at first sight appear to support the contention that co-evolution always leads to reduced pathogenicity, it remains the case that within any individual susceptible rabbit, or small population of susceptible rabbits, the more transmissible strains of myxoma virus (in this case, the more virulent and pathogenic strains) will always outcompete the less transmissible, less pathogenic strains.

The relationship between myxoma virus and wild rabbit populations today appears to be fairly stable – the rabbit population in the UK is currently about 40% of that in the 1950s – with smaller populations of rabbits existing in dynamic equilibrium with moderately virulent viruses.

The important point is that selection pressure acted to maximise R_0, requiring an evolutionary 'trade-off' between infectious period and pathogenicity, the balance of which will depend on the life histories of the parasite and its host in any particular environment.

of Europe the principal vectors appear to be mosquitoes, while in the UK, myxoma virus is primarily transmitted by fleas. In both situations the vector acquires the virus by feeding through infected skin. The virus survives on the mouthparts of the vector and is transmitted to a naïve host. As there is no biological interaction with the vector, viral survival depends on its ability to persist in the environment. Myxoma virus is a particularly robust virus, as are many poxviruses. It remains infective for many months both in the environment and on the mouthparts of the flea, while the mammalian host remains infectious for only a few weeks. Not all arthropod-borne infections are transmitted in a merely mechanical manner. In some cases transmission may be reliant on interactions between the vector and the microparasite. For example, when some species of flea feed on rodents infected with the plague bacillus (*Yersinia pestis*), the bacilli colonize the flea's proventriculus, where they replicate (15). Eventually, perhaps after feeding on several other rodents, the accumulation of bacteria at this site obstructs the flea's intestinal tract. Although the infected flea continues to feed despite the obstruction, ingested blood is regurgitated back into the vertebrate host, taking with it many bacteria.

Tick-borne infections differ fundamentally from those that are insect-borne because of differences in their feeding behaviour. The period between feeding on different individual hosts is greatly extended for many tick-borne infections. While most insects, particularly flies and mosquitoes, may feed on a number of hosts within a very short period, the life cycle of ticks prohibits such events. Hard ticks generally feed on three different hosts before completing their life cycle, and usually only on a single host during each instar, while the period between feeds can be several months. Recent studies on the tick *I. ricinus* suggest that questing nymphs and adults can survive for up to 12 months post moult, and that generally there is only one cohort of ticks recruited into the population each year. In such a situation it is obvious that for a microparasite to persist within a population, it must be able to survive within the tick for several months and, as such, transmission of tick-borne infections is almost invariably biological rather than mechanical. After feeding, excretion of waste products from the tick is rapid, and those microparasites unable to infect the tissues of the tick will also be excreted. The ability of microparasites to survive the moult and diapause that ticks undergo after each blood meal is termed trans-stadial transmission. *Borrelia burgdorferi* spirochaetes survive in the midgut of the tick, where they remain until the tick feeds on another host. At this stage they migrate to the tick salivary glands from where they can potentially infect the vertebrate host. The environment within a tick is vastly different to that within a mammal or bird but one way in which spirochaetes overcome this is by expressing different proteins, depending on their environment. While in the midgut of a resting tick, they primarily express outer surface protein A (OspA). If resident in a feeding tick, they down-regulate OspA and up-regulate outer surface protein C (OspC) as they migrate to the salivary glands. Spirochaetes continue to express Osp C during the initial stages of infection in the host. Conversely, when uninfected ticks acquire spirochaetes the bacteria up-regulate OspA, which appears to be important in binding the spirochaete to the midgut wall (see Chapter 9).

Some tick-borne infections are also transmitted transovarially and, in such cases, vertebrates may be more important as hosts for the vector rather than hosts to the infectious agent. Transmission of *Rickettsia rickettsii* (a member of the spotted fever group) from adult female *Dermacentor variabilis* to eggs and subsequently larvae can approach 100% efficiency under laboratory conditions, though figures of 30–50% appear to be more representative of those seen in nature. There is also some evidence that infection with *R. rickettsii* can have a

detrimental effect on the ticks themselves. Despite this, it appears that transovarial transmission may be more important in perpetuating infection in nature than the acquisition of the organism from rickettsaemic hosts, as rickettsaemia in mammalian hosts is generally short lived.

CONCLUSION

This chapter has introduced some of the concepts, often still being debated, about the ecological mechanisms that enable microparasites to persist in wild animal populations, and it has also provided explanations for some of the differences in the epidemiology and pathogenicity of arthropod-borne infections in wildlife compared with domestic animals and human beings. It is vital to understand the ecology of arthropod-borne infections in their reservoir hosts if we are to control these infections in accidental hosts such as domestic animals and human beings.

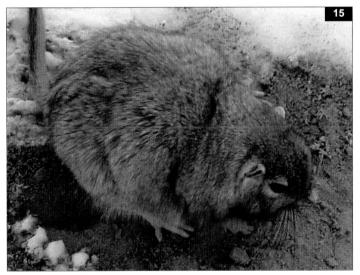

15 Giant gerbils (*Rhombomys opimus*) in Kazakhstan are important reservoir hosts for plague. Infection in other species occurs as a result of increases in the abundance of these giant gerbils.
(Photo courtesy of M Begon)

3 Interaction of the host immune system with arthropods and arthropod-borne infectious agents

Michael Day

INTRODUCTION

The transmission of infectious agents by haemophagous arthropods involves a unique three-way interaction between arthropod, microorganism and the host immune system. The aim of the arthropod in this interaction is to obtain a blood meal, using basic mechanisms that are relatively conserved between arthropod species. These include penetration of the host epidermal barrier and the secretion of a range of vasoactive and anticoagulant molecules that encourage local blood flow and permit uptake of the uncoagulated blood meal. Additionally, there is modulation of the local cutaneous immune and inflammatory responses by potent arthropod-derived molecules that are injected into the feeding site. This modulation may extend to influencing the immune response in regional lymphoid tissue and the systemic immune system and acting to prevent rejection of the arthropod, particularly those that require prolonged attachment to the host (i.e. ticks).

This manipulation of the host dermal micro-environment by infected arthropods also provides an advantage to microorganisms by creating an optimum environment for their transmission and the establishment of infection (16). This is exemplified by the persistence of infectious agents at the site of injection by ticks, which permits the infection of naïve ticks in the absence of systemic infection of the host ('saliva-activated transmission' [see Chapter 2]) (17). Additionally, the presence of organisms within an arthropod may modify its behaviour. For example, *Borrelia*-infected ticks have altered questing behaviour, which provides them with an advantage in terms of acquiring their target host. In contrast, *Leishmania*-infected sandflies also have modified feeding behaviour, but here the advantage is to the microorganism rather than the arthropod. The plug of *Leishmania* parasites within the proventriculus interferes with the intake of blood, making it necessary for the

sandfly to probe the host dermis more frequently. Such interactions are likely a result of the prolonged co-evolution of arthropods and the microorganisms that they carry.

The infectious agents transmitted by arthropods produce disease by a complex pathogenesis that may in part involve secondary immune-mediated phenomena. Both arthropod and microorganism may be involved in manipulating the host immune system to induce these sequelae to infection.

Unravelling of these complex pathways provides an insight into potential stages at which immunological control of the organism or the vector may be achieved. These mechanisms have been largely defined in experimental systems with a range of tick and fly species, but there have been limited studies in dogs and there are no reported studies of the interaction of ticks or flies with the immune system of cats. In contrast, the interaction of fleas with the canine and feline immune system is an area of continuing investigation, but these studies address the nature of salivary allergens rather than the ability of the flea to transmit pathogens to the host. The application of molecular technology to the study of the host-arthropod-microbe interaction will provide rapid advances in the future. The ability to sequence the complete genomes of both arthropods and microorganisms, coupled with studies of functional genomics and proteomics, will revolutionize this field.

This chapter will focus on relatively well characterized interactions of the mammalian immune system with ticks and sandflies, and the microorganisms transmitted by these arthropods. The potential for vaccination as a means of control of arthropod infestation and disease transmission will be addressed. Finally, the interaction of arthropod-borne microbes with the host immune system and the induction of secondary immune-mediated disease as part of the pathogenesis of infection will be discussed.

16 Effects of arthropod saliva on host biology. As part of the feeding process, haemophagous arthropods inject saliva into the host dermal microenvironment. Arthropod saliva mediates a range of local effects including vasodilation, inhibition of haemostasis and inhibition of host inflammatory and immune responses. In the case of ticks, there is also salivary transmission of infectious agents.

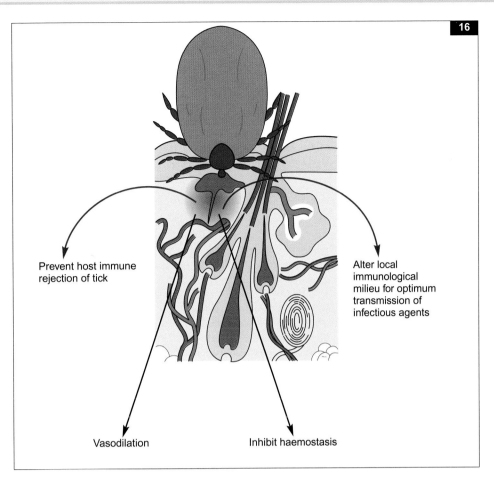

Prevent host immune rejection of tick

Alter local immunological milieu for optimum transmission of infectious agents

Vasodilation

Inhibit haemostasis

17 Saliva-activated transmission. In 'saliva-activated transmission' an arthropod injects an infectious agent into the host dermis. This agent persists at this location, likely due to inhibition of the host immune response by salivary molecules. For example, the saliva of some ticks inhibits the anti-viral effects of interferon and permits local replication of tick-transmitted virus. The persistent microbe may be taken up by uninfected arthropods that take a blood meal from the site, and this occurs in the absence of systemic viral infection. This mechanism has also been demonstrated for transmission of *Borrelia* that may be taken up by uninfected ticks prior to systemic spread of infection.

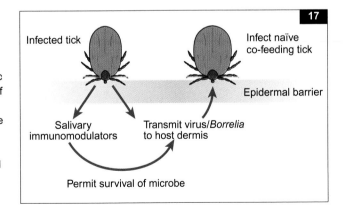

Infected tick

Infect naïve co-feeding tick

Epidermal barrier

Salivary immunomodulators

Transmit virus/*Borrelia* to host dermis

Permit survival of microbe

THE TICK–HOST INTERFACE: TICK MODULATION OF HOST BIOLOGY

Ticks have evolved specialized mechanisms that make them particularly effective haemophagous parasites, and the majority of these mechanisms are related to the secretion of a range of salivary proteins. The composition of tick salivary proteins has been studied biochemically. There is broad conservation in the range of molecules (by molecular weight) over several tick species and specific molecules are induced in the early stages of feeding. In several tick species, clear differences in the composition of male and female tick saliva have been demonstrated. In fed *Rhipicephalus appendiculatus*, specific novel proteins appear in haemolymph and then in saliva, suggesting that some inducible salivary antigens are obtained from haemolymph in this tick.

Tick cement

The action of tick mouthparts and deposition of 'cement' creates a firm attachment of tick to host that permits prolonged feeding and transmission of infectious agents. A 90 kDa salivary protein that is conserved amongst tick species and maximally secreted during the first two days of feeding has been suggested to be a cement component. A 29 kDa protein from *Haemaphysalis longicornis* has been cloned and sequenced and it has been proposed that this is also a cement component. Immunisation of rabbits with the recombinant 29 kDa protein confers protection.

Salivary anticoagulants

A continual flow of blood is required from the tick attachment site into the tick gut. This is achieved by the production of a range of anticoagulant salivary molecules that are injected into the feeding site. For example, apyrase is an inhibitor of ADP-induced platelet aggregation produced by many haemophagous parasites. *Amblyomma americanum* saliva inhibits Factor Xa and thrombin, and saliva from *R. appendiculatus* contains an anticoagulant that increases in concentration throughout feeding. Two anticoagulants have been characterized in the saliva of *Ixodes ricinus*: an antithromboplastin (ixodin) and a thrombin inhibitor (ixin).

Salivary osmoregulation and control of secretion

In addition to producing cement and anticoagulant molecules, the tick salivary gland also functions in osmoregulation. Excess fluid from an ingested blood meal is re-secreted to the host via tick saliva, and in free-living ticks the salivary gland functions in absorption of water vapour from the air. Tick salivary tissue undergoes hypertrophy and duct dilation during feeding and secretion is under neurological control. Nitric oxide may mediate duct dilation and dopamine has been shown to be an important neurotransmitter in this respect.

Salivary toxins

The salivary glands of a range of tick species secrete potent neurotoxins that interfere with the function of the neuromuscular synapse. This results in ascending motor paresis ('tick paralysis') and death may follow respiratory paralysis. A good example is the Australian tick *Ixodes holocyclus*, which produces the toxin holocyclin that may affect both dogs and cats.

Salivary anti-inflammatory molecules

Anti-inflammatory factors are also secreted into the host dermal microenvironment. These contribute to the ability of the tick to maintain prolonged attachment and, coincidentally, provide an optimum milieu for the transmission and establishment of infectious agents. Tick saliva contains prostaglandin E_2. This interacts with a PGE_2 receptor within the tick salivary gland, leading to secretion of further bioactive salivary proteins that may facilitate acquisition of a blood meal. Additionally, tick-derived PGE_2 may have an effector function when delivered to host tissue. Although considered unlikely to be a cause of immunosuppression, PGE_2 may have a local vasodilatory effect, thus enhancing delivery of the blood meal to the tick. Ticks cannot synthesize the prostaglandin precursor arachidonic acid, and must acquire this from the host. $PGF_{2\alpha}$, PGD_2 and PGB_2 have also been identified in saliva from ticks fed arachidonic acid.

The saliva of *Ixodes scapularis* has a kininase activity mediated by dipeptidyl carboxypeptidase. This inhibits bradykinin, therefore reducing local pain and inflammation and the likelihood of the host grooming-out the tick. The saliva of *R. appendiculatus* contains histamine-binding proteins that may compete with host histamine receptors for histamine and, therefore, reduce local inflammation. A novel, low molecular weight, anti-complement protein (isac) from the saliva of *I. scapularis* inhibits the alternative pathway of the complement cascade and inhibits generation of chemotactic C3a. In contrast, saliva from *Dermacentor andersoni* activates complement C5 to produce chemotactic effects.

Salivary immunomodulatory factors

The host immune response engendered by tick attachment has recently been discussed in terms of the Th1/Th2 paradigm, a fundamental immunological concept that has reshaped understanding of the host immune response to infectious agents. This model states that there are distinct functional subsets of CD4+ T lymphocytes that mediate either humoral or cell-mediated immunity. The humoral effects (type 2 immunity) are mediated by Th2 CD4+ T lymphocytes that produce the cytokines IL-4, IL-5, IL-6, IL-10 and IL-13. In contrast, cell-mediated immunity (type 1 immunity) is driven by the effects of Th1 CD4+ T cells that produce IL-2 and IFNγ (**18**). These two T cell subsets are counter-regulatory, so in some situations immune responses may become polarized towards a dominant humoral or cell-mediated response (**19**).

The two T cell subsets have a common precursor (a Th0 CD4+ T cell that produces a mixed cytokine profile). This requires particular activation signals to drive differentiation towards the mature Th1 or Th2 phenotype. These signals are largely derived from the antigen-presenting cell (APC) that activates the antigen-specific T lymphocyte. The nature of the APC signalling is determined by the binding of conserved molecular sequences (often derived from microbes) known as 'pathogen-associated molecular patterns' (PAMPs), with one of a series of 'pattern recognition' receptors expressed by the APC. For example, many bacterial sequences will induce the APC to secrete IL-12, which drives the development of a Th1 dominated immune response (**20**). This model has been largely developed with experimental rodent systems, so whether it extends to other species such as humans and dogs is not yet entirely clear.

The immunomodulatory effects of tick saliva may be manifest as an altered balance in the nature of the T cell

18 Functional dichotomy of helper T lymphocytes. The Th1/Th2 paradigm defines two functional subpopulations of CD4$^+$ T lymphocyte that are derived from a common Th0 precursor. These cells are defined by their function, which in turn is determined by the profile of cytokines that each selectively produces. Th1 cells are responsible for cell-mediated immunity and provide B cell help for production of a restricted subclass of IgG (IgG2a in mice). Th2 cells mediate humoral immunity, providing B cell help for production of IgE, IgA and IgG1. Th1 and Th2 cells are mutually antagonistic of each other via the secretion of specific inhibitory cytokines that counteract the function of the opposing subset.

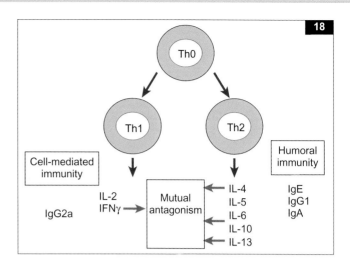

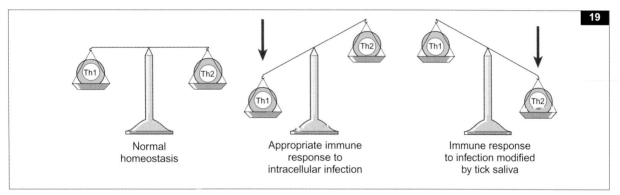

19 Immunomodulation by tick saliva. Th1 and Th2 cells may be normally thought of as being in balance. The immune response to particular types of antigen may disturb this balance and cause polarization of T cell function. In general, intracellular pathogens will only be effectively destroyed in the presence of strong Th1 cell-mediated immunity. However, the major effect of arthropod saliva is to alter the balance in favour of Th2 immunity, which favours replication of the pathogen.

20 Induction of the adaptive immune response to pathogens. Induction of either Th1 or Th2 immune responses depends largely on signals delivered to the Th0 precursor by the dendritic antigen presenting cell (APC). Antigens derived from pathogens are taken up and processed by the APC into peptide fragments that associate with class II molecules of the major histocompatibility complex (MHC). This complex of class II peptide is expressed on the APC membrane. A range of conserved motifs expressed by infectious agents (PAMPs) bind to 'pattern recognition receptors' (including those of the Toll-like receptor family) expressed on the APC. This induces dendritic cell maturation with further expression of MHC class II and co-stimulatory molecules (CD80/86).

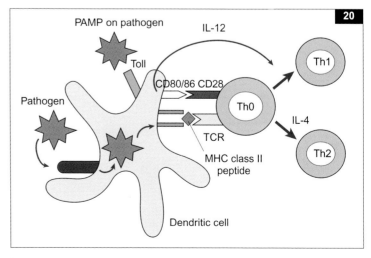

Additionally, the interaction with Toll-like receptor induces expression of cytokines such as IL-12 that selectively induces the Th1 subset. By contrast, IL-4 is required for Th2 activation but it is not known whether this cytokine may be regulated by Toll-like receptors.

response engendered by tick-derived or microbe-derived antigens. This altered balance is best detected by assessing the profile of cytokines produced by the activated T cells. These properties of tick saliva have been demonstrated by incorporation of *I. ricinus* salivary gland extract (SGE) into *in vitro* cell culture systems (**21**). A range of other immunomodulatory effects of *I. ricinus* SGE has also been shown, including reduction of cytotoxic function by activated murine NK cells and reduction of the ability of lipopolysaccharide (LPS)-stimulated macrophages to produce nitric oxide.

Similar studies have shown the immunomodulatory capacity of saliva from *Rhipicephalus sanguineus*. When lymph node cultures were established from tick-infested mice and stimulated with the mitogen Con A, there was reduced proliferation (relative to uninfested controls) and a distinct Th2 cytokine profile, with elevated IL-4, IL-10 and TGFβ, and reduced IL-2 and IFNγ production.

R. sanguineus saliva also inhibits Con A and antigen-driven proliferation and IL-2 production of murine splenic T cells.

In experimental rodent systems the immunomodulatory effects of tick saliva may be dependent on the strain of mouse used in the study. For example, exposure of C3H/HeJ mice to *Borrelia burgdorferi*-infected *I. scapularis* results in CD4[+] T cell proliferation and preferential Th2 immunity (raised IL-4, reduced IL-2, IFNγ), but these effects are not marked in Balb/c mice. These observations may underlie the susceptibility of C3H mice to borreliosis. In this experimental model, administration of recombinant Th1 cytokines to mice infested with *Borrelia*-infected *I. scapularis* led to a switch from Th2 to Th1 immunity (**22**). The effect of repeated infestation with uninfected *I. scapularis* on cytokine production by C3H/HeN and Balb/c mice has also been compared. Neither strain of

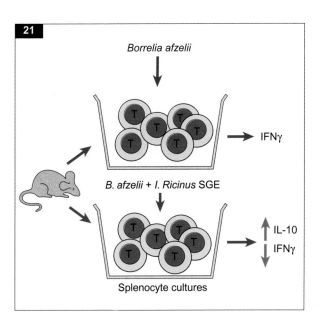

21 Tick saliva inhibits Th1 function. Murine spleen cells cultured *in vitro* in the presence of antigens such as *Borrelia afzelii* produce IFNγ that is released into the culture fluid and can be readily measured by techniques such as ELISA. However, when salivary gland extract from *Ixodes ricinus* is incorporated into the cultures, the cytokine profile changes to one of low IFNγ and high IL-10 production. Tick salivary molecules have switched this *in vitro* immune response from Th1 to Th2 in nature. (Experiments reported by Kopecky J *et al.* (1999) *Parasite Immunology* **21**, 351–356).

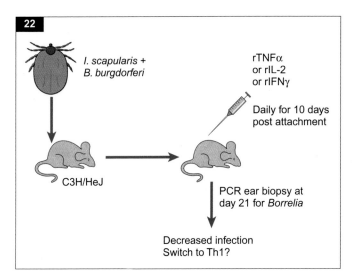

22 Immunosuppressive effect of tick saliva can be partially reversed by administration of Th1 cytokines. C3H mice were infested with *Ixodes scapularis* ticks that were infected with *Borrelia burgdorferi*. During the ten-day period following attachment of the ticks, different groups of mice were treated with recombinant cytokines that are associated with a Th1 immune response. At 21 days post attachment, biopsies of the ears were taken from the mice for determination of the *Borrelia* load by PCR. Mice treated with recombinant cytokine had reduced infection, suggesting that the Th2 inductive effects of tick saliva had been counteracted by enhancing the opposing Th1 response. (Experiments reported by Zeidner N *et al.* (1996) *Journal of Infectious Diseases* **173**, 187–195)

mouse became resistant to *I. scapularis* after four cycles of infestation but in both strains there was polarization of the cytokine profile to Th2 (**23**).

The immunosuppressive action of tick saliva has also been documented with *in vitro* studies of human cells. Saliva from fed *Dermacentor reticulatus* inhibits human NK cell function but saliva from unfed ticks does not. Similar but less potent inhibition of NK cells is mediated by SGE from *Amblyomma variegatum* and *Haemaphysalis inermis* but does not occur with SGE from *I. ricinus* or *R. appendiculatus*. SGE from *R. appendiculatus* reduces cytokine mRNA expression (IFNγ, IL-1, IL-5, IL-6, IL-7, IL-8, TNFα) by LPS-stimulated human peripheral blood lymphocytes (PBLs), and SGE from a range of Ixodid ticks can neutralize IL-8 and inhibit the neutrophil chemotaxis induced by this cytokine. Similarly, cattle infested with *Boophilus microplus* have altered *in vivo* immune function (reduced proportion of T cells in the blood and reduced antibody response to immunization with ovalbumin), and *B. microplus* saliva can suppress the *in vitro* response of bovine PBLs to the mitogen PHA. Experimental infestation of sheep with *Amblyomma variegatum* can influence the clinical course of *Dermatophilus congolensis*

infection at a separate skin site. Co-infected sheep have chronic, non-healing dermatophilosis, with chronic mononuclear cell infiltration of the dermis.

There have been limited studies of the interaction of tick saliva with the canine immune system. A series of studies from Japan have shown that infestation of dogs with *R. sanguineus* causes suppression of antibody production, neutrophil function and the response of blood lymphocytes to mitogens, and that *R. sanguineus* SGE can mimic these effects *in vitro*, suppressing both T and B lymphocyte subpopulations.

Some studies have addressed the molecular weight of the tick salivary immunosuppressive proteins by fractionation of saliva before inclusion in the *in vitro* systems described. The immunosuppressive activity of *R. sanguineus* saliva is mediated by proteins of under 10 kDa. Saliva from *Ixodes dammini* has an immunosuppressive activity of greater than 5 kDa and saliva from *Dermacentor andersoni* has two immunosuppressive components of molecular weights 36-43 and under 3 kDa.

Overall consideration of the experimental data on tick salivary immunosuppression permits the development of a hypothetical model for this effect and this is summarized in **24**.

23 Tick saliva induces Th2 activity through mechanisms other than IL-4 production. Balb/c mice were exposed to repeated cycles of infestation with *Ixodes ricinus* ticks. As expected, the immune system of the mice was switched towards Th2 responsiveness and the mice developed elevated levels of serum IgE. A parallel group of mice was treated with neutralizing monoclonal antibody to the cytokine IL-4 during the tick exposure; a group of mice with a targeted disruption to the IL-4 gene (IL-4 'knockout' mice, IL-4-/-) was also exposed to ticks. These latter two groups had reduced serum IgE but maintained the bias towards a Th2 immune response. This experiment suggests that IL-4 alone is not responsible for maintaining type 2 immunity. The failure to revert completely to type 1 immunity in these mice was mirrored by the fact that there was no difference in tick attachment or engorgement in the immunologically manipulated animals. (Experiments reported by Christie M et al. (1998) *Parasitological Research* **84**, 388–393)

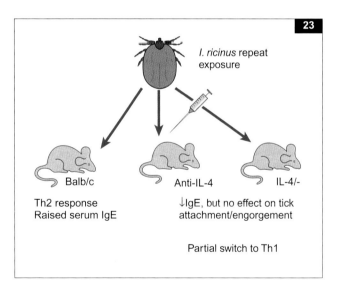

24 A model for the immunosuppressive effects of tick saliva. The salivary immunosuppressive proteins activate Th2 cells, with production of the key cytokine in this system, IL-10. The mechanism by which this selective activation occurs is unknown, but potentially it is either a direct effect on T cells or via the APC. IL-10 has a range of potent effects on macrophages, particularly in suppressing nitric oxide (NO) synthase. This in turn inhibits nitric oxide-dependent killing by macrophages of intracellular pathogens transmitted by the tick (e.g. *Ehrlichia, Rickettsia*). Moreover, the inhibition of macrophage activity leads to reduced IL-12 production and failure adequately to stimulate Th1 cells, which in turn results in reduced IFNγ production that further impairs macrophage activation.

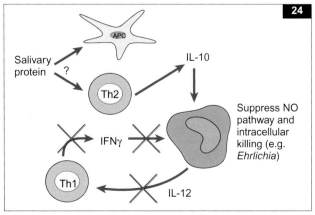

THE SANDFLY–HOST INTERFACE: SANDFLY MODULATION OF HOST BIOLOGY

In contrast to ticks, the interaction between host and haemophagous flies is relatively transient. Despite this, these insects also inject their hosts with powerful vasoactive, anticoagulant and immunomodulatory substances. The latter may not necessarily benefit an individual parasite but they will ensure that the host does not develop protective immunity and that it remains susceptible to the entire parasite population over a period of time. This section will focus on the sandfly vectors of leishmaniosis, as they are the most relevant to companion animal disease.

Salivary anticoagulants

The protein content of saliva is far greater in female sandflies and it increases over the first three days after emergence, which correlates with the fact that these flies do not usually bite hosts until after that time. Sandfly saliva has potent anticoagulant activity mediated by apyrase. SGE from the New World sandfly *Lutzomyia longipalpis* contains the powerful vasodilatory polypeptide maxadilan, whereas the saliva of Old World sandflies (e.g. *Phlebotomus papatasi*) mediates vasodilation via adenosine and 5'-AMP. The saliva of *L. longipalpis* also contains hyaluronidase, which may aid dispersal of other salivary molecules and of *Leishmania* within the host dermis.

Salivary immunomodulatory molecules

The saliva of the sandfly has potent immunoregulatory activity that is thought to underlie the ability of the saliva markedly to exacerbate *Leishmania* infection. SGE from *P. papatasi* causes a switch from a Th1 to Th2 response in mice infected with *Leishmania major* (e.g. increased IL-4 and reduced IFNγ in lymph nodes draining sites of experimental infection in the presence of SGE), and is inhibitory of macrophage function *in vitro*. These effects may be mediated by adenosine and 5'-AMP.

SGE from *L. longipalpis* inhibits presentation of *Leishmania* antigens by macrophages and thus suppresses antigen-specific lymphocyte proliferative responses and delayed type hypersensitivity (DTH). Macrophages co-cultured with *L. longipalpis* SGE were refractory to activation by IFNγ and unable to produce nitric oxide, hydrogen peroxide or proinflammatory cytokines (e.g. TNFα) – all necessary for destruction of the intracellular amastigotes. These effects are mediated by maxadilan, which has dual action as a vasodilator. Maxadilan has homology with mammalian pituitary adenylate cyclase-activating polypeptide (PACAP) and utilizes the receptor for this molecule that is expressed by macrophages. In an experimental murine model of *L. major* infection, the increased infectivity caused by sandfly saliva is due to maxadilan. The immunomodulatory effects of sandfly saliva may cause *in vitro* 'bystander suppression' of other immune responses.

HOST IMMUNE RESPONSE TO ARTHROPODS

This section discusses the protective host immune response to arthropods, as opposed to the ability of the arthropod to manipulate host immunity as has been described above. In general terms it appears that both humoral and cell-mediated immune responses are made to arthropod salivary proteins. The cutaneous immune response to tick attachment has been characterized in a number of species and is summarized in **25**. More is known about humoral immune responses than cellular responses, as these are more readily monitored. Several human epidemiological studies have shown that tick-exposed humans make anti-tick antibody responses, and these may correlate with the seroprevalence of infectious diseases in the same patients. For example, in a recent study of a Californian population, a significant correlation between seropositivity for *B. burgdorferi* and *I. pacificus* was reported. Similarly, antibody to a 24 kDa protein of *R. sanguineus* has been identified in the serum of dogs following two experimental infestations.

A series of studies has examined the comparative immune response to *R. sanguineus* made by dogs and guinea pigs. In these experiments, dogs were unable to develop resistance to infestation, whereas guinea pigs did become resistant. In one study, histopathological changes at tick attachment sites in each species were examined between four and 96 hours of attachment in primary, secondary or tertiary infestation. Although both species responded with a mononuclear cell infiltrate, the major difference was that dogs also responded with a neutrophilic infiltrate, whereas guinea pigs had a predominant eosinophil infiltrate, suggesting that this underlies resistance in the guinea pig. However, this study is at odds with the commonly accepted description of the histopathology of tick attachment sites in the dog, which includes a granulomatous inflammation and an eosinophil response (**26**). This may in part reflect the kinetics of the host response, as most skin biopsies collected in a clinical setting will be from tick bite reactions of greater than 96 hours duration. Other factors that may account for this discrepancy include the species and strain of tick, and whether the tick is infected with microorganisms.

In a similar study, the intradermal skin test response to an *R. sanguineus* extract was compared in naïve and infested dogs, and naïve and infested guinea pigs. Infested dogs developed a strong immediate reaction but infested guinea pigs had both immediate and delayed reactions. Control animals had no significant response. This provides evidence that cell-mediated immunity is one factor important for tick elimination and that this may be lacking in *R. sanguineus*-infested dogs. Resistance to *I. scapularis* has also been studied in the dog using a repeat infestation model. Tick performance parameters decreased with increasing exposure, suggesting the development of a protective immune response.

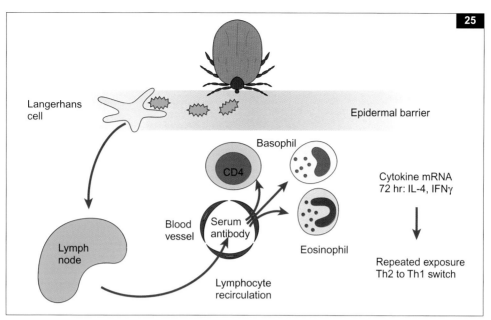

25 The host immune response to arthropods. The infested host will mount an immune response to arthropods, and repeated exposure can induce resistance in some individuals. In the case of ticks, the immune response will predominantly be directed against the injected salivary antigens. These will be captured by dendritic APCs in the epidermis (Langerhans cells) or dermis, and carried to the regional draining lymph nodes where activation of antigen-specific T and B lymphocytes occurs. Serum antibody specific for the salivary antigens will be induced. Antigen-specific T cells will be recruited back to the site of tick exposure via the interaction of lymphocyte homing receptors and the vascular addressins expressed by the endothelium of vessels in the tick attachment site. Locally produced cytokines and chemokines will recruit other leucocytes, chiefly eosinophils and basophils, to this dermal location. The nature of the dermal immune response will initially (up to 72 hours) reflect the immunomodulatory properties of the tick saliva (Th2 dominated), with mRNA encoding both IL-4 and IFNγ found at the attachment sites. With time the cytokine profile will switch and the site will become Th1-dominated.

26 Histopathology of the tick attachment site. Skin biopsy from a tick attachment site on a dog. There is a central region of ulceration and necrosis that correlates with the site of attachment and production of the salivary cement substance. This is surrounded by a heavy infiltration of mixed mononuclear cells (including macrophages, lymphocytes and plasma cells) and eosinophils in this relatively chronic lesion. (Haematoxylin and eosin)

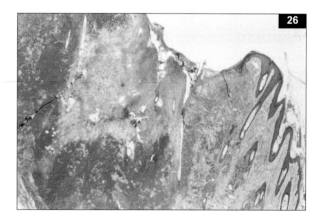

The immune response to the salivary proteins of sandfly saliva has been extensively studied in experimental models and it is clear that strong antibody and DTH responses can be made following the bite of uninfected sandflies, injection with SGE or with recombinant salivary proteins. However, despite numerous studies of the immune response to *Leishmania* in infected dogs, there have been no reported investigations of the response to sandfly saliva or the nature of the cutaneous lesions that might develop following the bite of these flies. Even less is known about how the immune system of the cat might respond to sandfly bites.

VACCINATION AGAINST ARTHROPODS

Vaccination against ticks

Vaccination strategies have been devised to limit tick infestation and, therefore, the transmission of tick-borne microbes. Additionally, there has been much research into the development of vaccines for the individual microbial agents themselves. Detailed discussion of the latter is beyond the scope of this review but will be covered in the individual chapters of this book.

Tick salivary cDNA libraries have been created and molecules of immunological relevance have been identified by screening the libraries expressed in vector systems with sera from immune animals. For example, a feeding-induced gene from *I. scapularis* (Salp 16) was cloned in this manner and recombinant Salp 16 produced. Although *I. scapularis* infested guinea pigs made high titred serum antibody to Salp 16, vaccination with the recombinant molecule did not protect from infestation.

Although there have been numerous such studies of candidate tick vaccines, only one recombinant product has been produced commercially. The vaccine for bovine *B. microplus* infestation contains the recombinant antigen Bm86 and induces antibodies in immunized cattle that mediate lysis of tick gut cells when ingested in a blood meal. The reduced tick burden and fecundity produced as a result allows decreased frequency of acaricide application to vaccinated animals. Some strains of *B. microplus* are resistant to the Bm86 vaccine but may be susceptible to a preparation containing the Bm95 recombinant antigen. Some tick-derived molecules may induce cross-protection against other tick species that carry homologous antigenic epitopes, and the Bm86 vaccine offers such cross-protection against at least two other tick species.

A recent study has examined the efficacy of vaccinating naïve dogs with salivary gland or midgut extracts of *R. sanguineus* before repeat experimental challenge seven and 21 days after the final vaccination. During these challenges there was reduced tick attachment (for both salivary and midgut vaccines), feeding period and engorgement weight (greatest with salivary vaccine) and fecundity (greatest with midgut vaccine). The observed greater efficacy of the gut extract may reflect the fact that the host is normally exposed to salivary antigens, and the tick may have developed means of suppressing the host response to such antigens during co-evolution. Moreover, a control group repeatedly exposed to *R. sanguineus* also showed transient reductions in these tick performance parameters, suggesting that dogs can develop spontaneous immunity to *R. sanguineus*. Immunization of dogs with gut extract of *R. sanguineus* in Freund's adjuvant was more effective than this extract adjuvanted in saponin, evidence for the importance of cell-mediated immunity in resistance of dogs to these ticks.

A similar study has been reported in cattle with *Hyalomma marginatum* extracts but in this instance immunity, induced by repeat infestation or salivary extract vaccination, was superior to vaccination with an intestinal extract of the tick. Vaccination of cattle with SGE of *Hyalomma anatolicum* in Freund's incomplete adjuvant can be enhanced by incorporation of the additional adjuvant effect of *Ascaris suis* extract into the vaccine. The *A. suis* extract enhances IgE responses and produces a greater immediate hypersensitivity skin test reaction in immunized calves.

Vaccination against sandflies

Vaccination against other arthropods has also been investigated as a potential control measure for the microbial infections they transmit. Mice experimentally infected with *Leishmania major* develop significantly more severe disease when co-injected with entire SGE or with synthetic maxadilan from *L. longipalpis*, suggesting that this latter molecule is responsible for the disease exacerbation caused by sandfly saliva. Vaccination with synthetic maxadilan induces a type 1 immune response and serum antibody specific for the molecule, and protects mice from experimental infection with *L. major*. The Old World sandfly *Phlebotomus papatasi* does not produce maxadilan, but pre-exposure to the bite of uninfected *Phlebotomus* confers resistance to infection with *L. major* with a strong DTH response, suggesting a similar effect with an alternative candidate protein. A recent study characterized nine salivary proteins from *P. papatasi* and demonstrated that a recombinant form of one of these (SP15) was able to induce strong DTH in mice and was protective when used as a vaccine against *L. major*.

A recent unpublished abstract reported an experimental study in dogs co-injected with *Leishmania* and sandfly SGE. Relative to controls that received only *Leishmania*, the test dogs developed clinical leishmaniosis several months earlier, which correlated with earlier demonstration of *Leishmania*-specific T cell proliferative responses and IL-4 production. The investigators suggested that this 'early onset' model of canine leishmaniosis would permit more rapid assessment of *Leishmania* vaccines in the dog model.

IMMUNE-MEDIATED SEQUELAE TO ARTHROPOD-TRANSMITTED INFECTIOUS DISEASE

The range of arthropod-transmitted pathogens that are the subject of this book have complex pathogenesis within the host. In broad terms, many of the clinical disease manifestations in leishmaniosis, babesiosis, ehrlichiosis, anaplasmosis, borreliosis, rickettsiosis, bartonellosis and hepatozoonosis are related to the interaction of the infectious agent with the host immune system. These clinical manifestations will be discussed in other chapters. It is suggested that the initial interaction of arthropod products with the host immune system may redirect host immunity to a state that is optimum for subsequent immune-mediated disease related to the microbe (27). In this respect, if arthropod salivary molecules are able to subvert the host immune system and create a 'switch' to type 2 (humoral) immunity, the

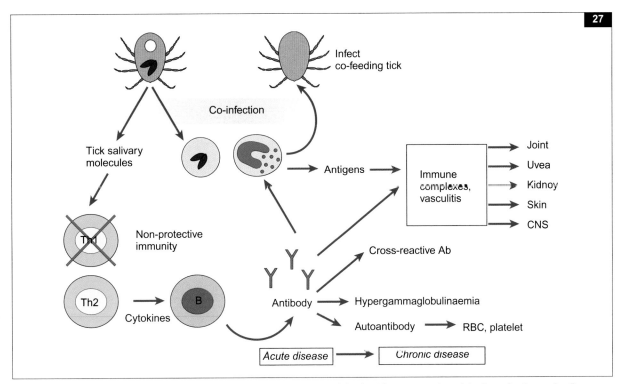

27 Summary of the interaction between arthropod, infectious agent and the host immune system. Injection of arthropod salivary molecules results in redirection of the host immune system to the Th2 phenotype, both locally within the dermis and within the regional draining lymph node. In rodent model systems this effect may also involve the systemic immune system. Salivary immunomodulation permits prolonged or repeated exposure to the arthropod and allows transmission of the arthropod-borne infectious agent (or agents in co-infections) and establishment of infection in the absence of a protective (type 1) immune response. Uninfected arthropods co-feeding at the site may acquire infection ('saliva-activated transmission'). The infectious agent may spread from the site of inoculation to produce parasitaemia and acute infectious disease. The bias towards Th2 immunity may also underlie the chronic, secondary, immune-mediated sequelae to infection. These include excessive B cell activation (hypergammaglobulinaemia), the formation of circulating immune complexes that may deposit within the microvasculature, and the induction of autoantibodies or antibodies that cross-react with microbial and self epitopes. (Redrawn after Shaw SE *et al.* (2001) *Trends in Parasitology* **17**, 74–80)

likelihood is that if an infectious agent is superimposed on the immune system in this state, there will be humoral immune-mediated sequelae. For example:

- Hyperglobulinaemia via polyclonal or monoclonal B cell activation (e.g. in leishmaniosis or monocytic ehrlichiosis).
- Induction of autoantibody (e.g. anti-erythrocyte in babesiosis, anti-platelet in ehrlichiosis and rickettsiosis, both autoantibodies in leishmaniosis) or induction of cross-reactive antibody by molecular mimicry between autoantigen and epitopes of the infectious agent (e.g. cross-reactivity of antibodies to neuroaxonal proteins and flagellin from *Borrelia*).
- Formation of circulating immune complexes of antibody and microbial or self antigen that may potentially lodge in capillary beds and cause local tissue pathology (e.g. uveitis, polyarthritis, vasculitis and glomerulonephritis that may occur in leishmaniosis).
- Granulomatous inflammatory aggregates of parasitized macrophages that are unable effectively to kill the intracellular microbe (e.g. dermal lesions in leishmaniosis).

Such effects may be further complicated when there is multiple co-infection with arthropod-transmitted infectious agents. This model of type 2 directed immunity is not all-encompassing, as type 1 (cell-mediated) effects do comprise part of the pathogenesis of such infections; for example, the mononuclear cell synovitis that occurs in borreliosis is T cell mediated and the specificity of these T cells has been characterized.

CONCLUSIONS

The attachment of an infected arthropod to a mammalian host creates a severe challenge to the host immune system. Host immunity to arthropods and arthropod-transmitted infectious agents is based on a cell-mediated (Th1) response, but arthropod salivary molecules are able to subvert host immunity to a dominant Th2 (humoral) form. This permits prolonged feeding by individual arthropods (ticks) or populations (sandflies) and transmission of infectious agents into an environment in which the host preferentially generates humoral immunity to the organism. This latter effect may underlie the range of immunopathogenic mechanisms that characterize arthropod-borne infections.

4 Laboratory diagnosis of arthropod-transmitted infections

Martin Kenny

INTRODUCTION

The arthropod-transmitted pathogens discussed in this book are generally difficult to cultivate *in vitro*, are often present in very low numbers in peripheral blood and the clinical signs they cause are very variable, as are the antibody responses they may evoke. The individual organisms are dealt with in detail in later chapters. This chapter gives an overview of the diagnostic tests used for determining infection with these agents.

'CLASSICAL' DIAGNOSTIC METHODS

Culture/propagation of pathogens

The arthropod-transmitted pathogens generally have exacting nutritional requirements, reflecting their intracellular or epicellular modes of existence, and are difficult to grow *in vitro*. In exceptional cases, where growth on synthetic, or semi-synthetic, media is possible, growth rates are very slow, with an attendant high risk of fungal or bacterial contamination despite rigorous aseptic technique.

Table 4 Components present in media for cultivation of some *Bartonella* and *Borrelia* species.

Bartonella species: **Columbia agar**	*Borrelia burgdorferi* (sensu stricto): **BSK medium**
Peptone	Glutamine
Trypteine	Proteose peptone, tryptone and yeastolate
Yeast extract	HEPES*
Heart infusion extract	Sodium citrate
Starch	Glucose
Sodium chloride	Sodium pyruvate
Agar	CMRL-1066 tissue culture medium
Whole horse blood	N-acetylglucosamine
	Magnesium chloride
	Gelatine
	Bovine serum albumin (Fraction V)
	Rabbit serum, inactivated

* N-2[hydroxyethyl]piperazine-N'-[2-ethanesulphonic acid]

Borrelia burgdorferi and certain *Bartonella* species (e.g. *B. henselae*) can be grown on media (*Table 4*). In both cases it can take a month between inoculation with clinical material and identification of visible growth, making culture inappropriate for diagnosis. Culture has the advantage of allowing analysis of relatively large sample volumes and it has high sensitivity. This is because a single organism in a millilitre of blood will give rise to a colony that can be used as the basis for more advanced tests. Ideally, several replicates of each sample should be inoculated to allow contamination and sensitivity issues to be addressed.

Microscopy

In the hands of experienced microscopists, some parasites may be definitively identified on the basis of their morphology (e.g. *Babesia divergens*), their cellular tropisms (e.g. *Ehrlichia canis* selectively infects monocytes; *Anaplasma platys* infects platelets; and *A. phagocytophilum* infects neutrophils), or their staining characteristics in peripheral blood smears (e.g. *Mycoplasma haemominutum* and *M. haemofelis*). However, a common problem encountered in pathology laboratories is the interpretation of suboptimally prepared blood smears. A checklist of considerations necessary in optimum smear preparation is included in *Table 5* (see p. 42).

Standard differential stains such as May Grünwald Giemsa work well in blood smears for large protozoan parasites, such as *Leishmania* species and *Babesia* species, and the multicellular aggregates (morulae) of *Ehrlichia* species. In order to view bacteria such as *Bartonella* or the rickettsias directly, more advanced staining methods such as the Warthin–Starry silver stain can be employed using suitably prepared biopsy material. However, these are relatively non-specific and results must be interpreted with caution.

For motile bacteria such as *Borrelia* species, darkfield microscopy, which utilizes a special condenser to direct light toward an object at an angle, rather than from below, may be used. Using this method, particles or cells are seen as light objects against a dark background. Darkfield microscopy or phase contrast microscopy may be used on fresh material (e.g. synovial fluid) to observe

Table 5 Making the perfect blood film.

- **Use EDTA as anti-coagulant.** EDTA gives superior preservation of host and parasite cell morphology.
- **Mix blood well (but gently) prior to making the film.**
- **Avoid delay in making the blood film.** Blood films should ideally be made within one hour of collecting the blood sample; even if the sample cannot be stained or examined, it is better if the film is prepared as soon as possible.
- **Avoid using too much blood.** The commonest problem. A tiny drop should be applied to the slide using an applicator or pipette tip.
- **Spread the film evenly.** Spread the blood drop using another glass slide. Touch the drop then draw the slide away at an angle of 30–40° in a smooth glide.
- **Air-dry the film as soon as possible.** Water-induced artefacts are reduced by rapid drying of the slide. Waving the slide vigorously, or using a flame or hair drier, are all effective, particularly in humid environments.
- **Keep staining solutions clean.** Stain sediment is a common problem in diagnosis of haemoplasmas and *Babesia* species. Stains should be filtered before use. Fresh stain and fixative solutions should be prepared regularly.
- **Use a coverslip.** Using a coverslip greatly enhances the visual image. It may be temporarily mounted with immersion oil.

(Dr P Irwin, personal communication)

organisms. Antibodies specific for particular pathogens, linked to fluorescent dyes, can be used in conjunction with a fluorescence microscope to detect organisms in blood smears or tissue sections.

Antibody-based methods (serology)

In general, exposure of mammals to complex non-self antigens (e.g. the surface components of a bacterium) results in the induction of an immune response. This response is characterized by the generation of antibody and/or cell-mediated immunity. Serology, in the context of this chapter, is the study of antibody responses to infectious agents.

The nature and scale of the humoral immune response can give valuable information about host exposure to an infectious agent but is less helpful in assessing active infection or in quantifying the infectious load. Some of the more relevant methods involved in the detection of antibodies with specificities for particular organisms or proteins are described below. Serum (or plasma for some applications) should be separated as soon as possible from the blood clot or cell pellet to minimize the chance of haemoglobin contamination, which may interfere with some applications. Gel tubes provide an efficient means of obtaining clear, stable serum.

The kinetics of the humoral response to many pathogenic organisms have been described in detail and should be understood if logical conclusions are to be drawn from serological testing. The response to sequential challenge with antigen in terms of antibody class and concentration is illustrated (**28**). The nature of the response is determined by the number of exposures to the antigen. Following the initial exposure, a second or third exposure (or, more realistically, continued exposure) gives rise to more rapid induction of IgG compared to IgM, which predominates in the early stages of infection.

Infection, or 'challenge', with a pathogen to which the animal has had no previous exposure evokes a weak IgM response after one week, and a gradually increasing IgG

response, which peaks after about 14 days. Measuring antibody levels in an animal with acute-onset disease, such as babesiosis, would thus give little useful diagnostic information. For more chronic and persistent infections, such as that caused by *Ehrlichia canis*, measuring antibody levels may be more clinically useful, particularly when correlated with the epidemiology of the disease in question. For example, low levels of antibody to *Rickettsia rickettsii* may be incidental in animals that are, or have been, resident in endemic areas, but may be significant in animals that have returned to a non-endemic area after a short visit to an endemic area.

The production of antibodies is an idiosyncratic process, varying in both scale and specificity between animals depending upon age, health status and genetic background. The best way of assessing whether seroconversion to a particular pathogen has occurred is to analyse paired samples collected two to three weeks apart. A rising antibody titre suggests a recent and, therefore, clinically significant infection, especially if supported by appropriate clinical signs. An alternative method for determining recent infection is to measure

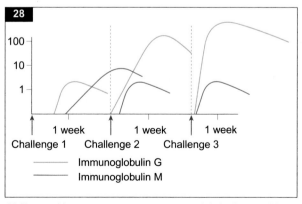

28 Humoral immune responses to sequential challenge with antigen in terms of antibody class and concentration.

antigen-specific IgM concentrations. This is technically more demanding and may give spurious results where high concentrations of IgG are present in a sample. IgM concentrations are particularly useful in cases where diseases are endemic and a high proportion of the population may have antigen-specific IgG.

Antibodies recognize small (~12 amino acid) regions of antigenic proteins as well as larger structural ('conformational') determinants. Because of the modular way in which biological polymers are 'designed', it is quite often the case that two unrelated proteins will share structural or protein sequence motifs. This leads to the phenomenon of cross-reaction whereby antibodies may recognize molecules other than those that originally generated the immune response. Whilst this is an excellent strategy in evolutionary terms, for experimental purposes it can be frustrating, leading to false-positive results. For example, if one looks for antibodies against the agent of Lyme disease, *Borrelia burgdorferi sensu stricto*, one must ensure that exposure to related, non-pathogenic spirochaetes, or to vaccinal antibodies (e.g. to *Leptospira* species), will not be detected by the assay.

A number of the arthropod-transmitted pathogens specifically target cells involved in the immune response; for example, *Leishmania* species multiply in macrophages and *Ehrlichia canis* has a tropism for monocytes. These organisms frequently dysregulate antibody production, causing the production of large quantities of non-specific IgG (monoclonal or polyclonal gammopathies). These are mostly non-functional antibodies with respect to the organism, although they may be autoreactive and thus contribute to pathology. However, they may also cause interference in diagnostic serological methods. The presence of gammopathy can be a useful clue when investigating more chronic arthropod-borne infections; indeed, IgG 'spikes' on serum electrophoresis are sometimes the first results to raise suspicion as to the possibility of an infectious agent being responsible for disease. To complicate matters further, certain arthropod-borne pathogens are actively immunosuppressive (e.g. *Anaplasma phagocytophilum*) and infected animals may show spuriously low antibody levels despite active infection.

Despite the caveats described above, antibody-based diagnostic tests are widely used commercially and in practice. Five methods are commonly used for detecting antibodies in serum samples.

Enzyme-linked immunosorbent assay (ELISA)

ELISA uses the principle that proteins can be induced to adhere irreversibly to certain plastic surfaces. Immobilized antigen can be used to 'trap' complementary antibodies in a serum sample. The amount of antibody in the sample is determined by using a series of serum dilutions and assessing the limit at which the detection signal is statistically indistinguishable from that of background 'noise'. Binding of this primary serum antibody to the immobilized antigen is detected using a secondary antibody, produced against purified immunoglobulins of the species from which the test serum came, which has been conjugated to an enzyme (usually alkaline phosphatase or horseradish peroxidase). After a series of incubation steps, a visualization reagent is added, which contains a chromogenic substrate for the conjugated enzymes. The reaction is stopped after a set period of time and the last serum dilution resulting in an unequivocally detectable amount of colour is determined spectrophotometrically. The titre of antibody is defined as the inverse of this last detectable dilution (e.g. a serum sample titrating to a dilution of 1:2,000 is quoted as having an antibody titre of 2,000). The processes involved are depicted (**29**).

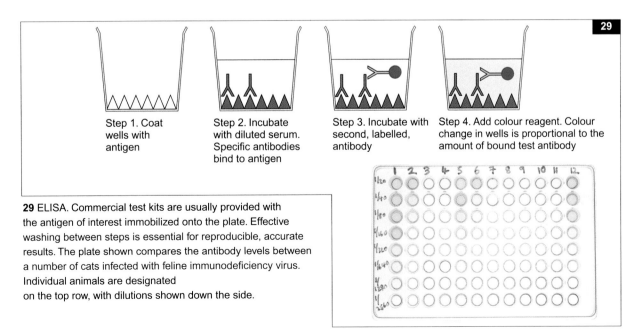

Step 1. Coat wells with antigen

Step 2. Incubate with diluted serum. Specific antibodies bind to antigen

Step 3. Incubate with second, labelled, antibody

Step 4. Add colour reagent. Colour change in wells is proportional to the amount of bound test antibody

29 ELISA. Commercial test kits are usually provided with the antigen of interest immobilized onto the plate. Effective washing between steps is essential for reproducible, accurate results. The plate shown compares the antibody levels between a number of cats infected with feline immunodeficiency virus. Individual animals are designated on the top row, with dilutions shown down the side.

ELISAs have become the preferred format for determining the presence of antibodies against pathogens from which antigens are freely available; that is, for pathogens which are relatively easy to cultivate or from which protein antigens have been identified, cloned and expressed as recombinant proteins. The attraction of ELISA technology is that it can be performed in a microtitre plate format, is easy to automate and produces numerical, objective data. These features make ELISA ideal for studies where the immune status of large numbers of animals is to be determined, as in vaccine trials or sero-epidemiological surveys. If the appropriate second antibodies are used, IgM or IgG (or both) can be measured in a sample.

The ELISA format can also be used to detect antigen in samples if high affinity antibodies are available with which to coat the plates (the capture antibody) and to detect bound antigen (the visualization antibody). Monoclonal antibodies (or fragments) are generally used in this context. For example, antigen ELISA is a sensitive and specific tool for diagnosing *Dirofilaria immitis* (heartworm) infection. In some instances, multiple pathogens can be tested for simultaneously in a single module such as the Snap 3Dx™ kit, which allows simultaneous testing for the presence of antibodies to *Ehrlichia canis* and *Borrelia burgdorferi* and heartworm antigen in a blood sample.

Immunofluorescent assay (IFA)

Where culture of organisms is difficult, or not advisable due to safety concerns, another serological technique may be used. In fluorescent antibody tests (FAT), organisms may be detected in infected cells or tissues of a patient (direct testing) or, more commonly, the presence of serum antigen-specific antibodies may be determined using an infected cell or tissue substrate (indirect testing [IFAT]). The robustness of the antibody molecule is used to provide a reagent that can discriminate between closely related protein molecules. In IFAT, infected cells, usually derived from tissue culture, are fixed onto microscope slides or microtitre plates. A procedure similar to that described for ELISA (see p. 43) is then employed to determine if a serum sample contains antibodies against the particular pathogen (30). However, instead of using a chromogenic conjugate, the second antibody is labelled with a dye molecule (e.g. fluorescein or Texas Red), which fluoresces under light of a particular wavelength. Samples containing antibodies cause the organisms within infected cells to glow brightly when viewed with a fluorescence microscope. This method is widely used in studying antibody status to *Leishmania* and *Babesia* species. As with ELISA, the amount of antibody in a sample is determined by limiting dilution and the results are given as a titre.

A similar but less sensitive method, the direct fluorescent antibody test, involves incubating test tissue sections or blood smears with a high affinity, fluorescently-labelled antibody, often a monoclonal antibody, specific for the pathogen in question. This method is used to detect pathogens such as *A. phagocytophilum*, where the number of infected cells may be low. Under fluorescent light, the infected cells are immediately apparent.

Agglutination-based tests

The multivalency of antigen-binding sites on antibody molecules (two for IgG; ten for IgM) allows them to cross-link macromolecular structures (**31**). This cross-linking, or agglutination, is clearly visible because the initial homogeneous suspension of carrier particles (e.g. latex beads or tanned red blood cells) becomes turbid as the individual particles aggregate. This test can be performed on any solid surface and can use inexpensive carriers such as latex beads. The agglutination occurs rapidly at room temperature. Agglutination tests provide a rapid, simple method for detection of pathogen exposure or for determination of post-vaccination titres. Because the test relies on a universal property of antibodies, it can be used for all species suspected of seroconversion to a pathogen. Agglutination tests are also valuable because they can detect antigen or antibody, provided that target material is available to coat the beads.

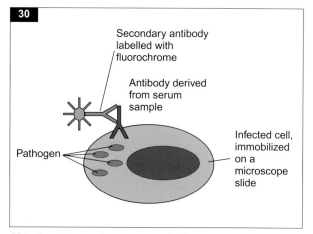

30 Indirect immunofluorescent antibody assay. Infected cells are immobilized onto an inert substrate. Serum (serially diluted in a number of tests performed in parallel) is then applied. After washing unbound antibodies away, an appropriate purified antibody bound to a fluorescent dye is added. An intense fluorescence is observed in tests containing antibody concentrations above a certain threshold.

A sensitive and specific latex bead agglutination test has been validated for investigating human leishmaniosis in rural communities in Sudan. It uses latex beads coated with high affinity, purified IgG specific for *Leishmania* and has been developed to detect urinary antigen. A comparison of IFA, agglutination and immunomigration methods (see below) for detecting *Leishmania* antibodies showed that agglutination, despite its simplicity, had the highest sensitivity.

Rapid immunomigration tests

A number of 'in-practice' tests have been developed that allow rapid determination of an animal's immune status with respect to particular infectious agents. A number of the tests available for arthropod-borne pathogens are variants of the ELISA technique described earlier (e.g. ImmunoComb™ and SNAP™ tests). A different method, known as rapid immunomigration (RIM), is used in tests such as the WITNESS™ system. This method is a passive chromatography system where animal serum is added to a membrane containing gold-labelled antigens in solution. Any specific antibodies in the serum bind to the antigen and the resultant antibody-antigen complexes move along the test strip until they reach a matrix that precipitates the complex. Antibody-antigen complexes appear as a pink line in this precipitation zone. The kit comes with appropriate positive and negative controls and is semi-quantitative. In an alternative method, the test kit contains labelled antibodies to a particular antigen, allowing antigen in a sample to be detected. An example is shown (**32**).

Immunoblotting ('western blotting' or 'dot blotting')

ELISA, IFA, agglutination and RIM tests generally employ a complex mixture of antigens such as cellular homogenates to capture reactive antibodies. Therefore, when a positive result is obtained, minimal information is obtained about the antigen-antibody binding events occurring in the test. For example, an animal may have antibodies that non-specifically adhere to a component of the plastic microtitre plate in an ELISA test, and the subsequent reaction would be read as a positive reaction to a pathogen. Alternatively, antibodies to common environmental antigens may cross-react with components of the antigen mixture used in the test of interest, producing false seropositivity. It is possible to circumvent these problems using pathogen-specific recombinant proteins that are also relevant to the disease process.

31 Agglutination-based assay. Diagrammatic representation of the first stage of the agglutination process. The bivalency of the IgG molecule allows it to cross-link relatively large particles. The cross-linking becomes apparent as the particles cohere and the original solution becomes heterogeneous. This is seen as an increased rate of precipitation of the inert carrier. IgM molecules are pentavalent and are much more efficient 'agglutinins'.

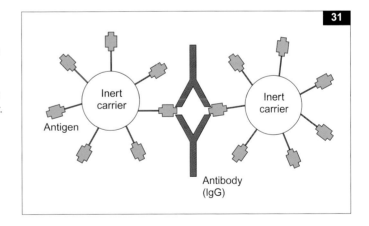

32 Rapid immunomigration. The slide shows a positive result for *Borrelia* serology. Serum is added to well A; a pink band in window B indicates a positive result. The band in window C is a positive control that shows that the test is functioning correctly.

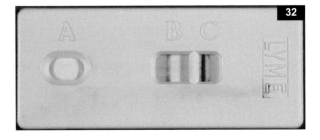

An alternative method for visualizing antigen-antibody interactions is immunoblotting. A complex mixture of antigens (best applied to proteins) is separated, according to molecular weight, with denaturing, sodium dodecyl sulphate polyacrylamide gel electrophoresis (SDS-PAGE). The proteins are then transferred and immobilized on an inert membrane (e.g. nitrocellulose). Unoccupied protein-binding sites are then 'blocked' and the membrane is 'probed' with a primary antibody against the antigen(s) of interest, as in ELISA and IFAT tests. An enzyme-labelled second antibody is then used to detect binding of primary antibody; addition of a specific substrate solution (giving a precipitate in this case, rather than the soluble ELISA product) then allows visualization of antigenic bands. The molecular weights of these bands can be determined by reference to a mixture of known molecular weight proteins separated on the same gel (33). An alternative to chromogenic substrates are those substrates that emit light that can then be detected on photographic film; this chemiluminescent system is more versatile and can give enhanced sensitivity. The results from clinical samples can be compared to patterns seen in confirmed infections and they add weight to the credibility of ELISA tests. The use of immunoblotting has become established in the diagnosis of Lyme disease, where ELISA results have a significant false-positive rate and where vaccinal antibodies (which are detected by ELISA) can be distinguished from naturally induced antibodies.

Xenodiagnosis

The difficulty in cultivating many tick-transmitted organisms can be circumvented by feeding laboratory reared, 'clean', arthropod vectors (ticks, fleas or flies) on presumptively infected blood. Under optimal environmental conditions, organisms will multiply rapidly in the appropriate vector and can be easily visualized by plain immunofluorescence-enhanced microscopy. This amplification method has been used to advantage in the diagnosis of human *Trypanosoma cruzi* infection. Triatomid bug nymphs are allowed to feed on people with presumed chronic Chagas' disease. On engorgement (20–30 minutes), the bugs are removed and kept under controlled conditions for 20–30 days. At this time, motile trypanosomes are detected by dark field microscopy in the faeces and body contents of the bug if the person on whom it fed was infected.

DNA-BASED DIAGNOSTIC METHODS

The genome of a pathogen contains all the information required to produce the proteins and RNA molecules that it requires to successfully propagate itself. The sum of the gene expression that takes place within a pathogen is expressed as the phenotype. Looked at globally, the DNA sequences of the genes that are essential for life are quite similar between apparently unrelated organisms. However, the small, subtle changes in DNA sequences that occur due to random mutation, and which offer a selective advantage, or are selectively neutral over geological time frames, differentiate one pathogen from another. In the last twenty years a revolution has taken place in our ability to dissect, analyse and understand genomes. This section describes how these advances have been applied to the identification of previously difficult-to-detect organisms.

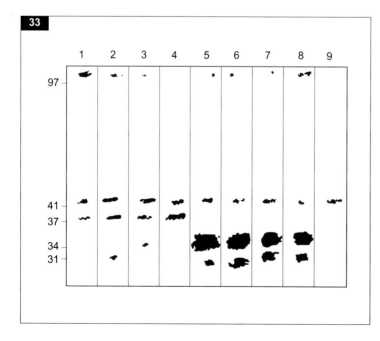

33 Immunoblot analysis to compare the antibody profiles of dogs that have been naturally infected or vaccinated with *Borrelia burgdorferi* (simplified for clarity); all dogs positive by standard ELISA. Proteins from sonicated *B. burgdorferi* were separated by sodium dodecyl sulphate polyacryla-mide gel electrophoresis then transferred to nitrocellulose. Strips of membrane were then probed with sera from naturally infected (1–4) or vaccinated animals (5–8). Serum from an animal from a Lyme disease-free area was used as a control (9). It can be seen that antibodies to antigens of 97 kDa and 41 kDa are common to both groups of dogs. Antibodies to the 34 kDa and 31 kDa proteins (OspB and OspA repectively) are much more pronounced in the vaccinated animals. The 41 kDa band (flagellin) is shared with other spirochaetes including *Leptospira* species, perhaps explaining the cross-reactive antibody seen in the negative control. In this example, 37 kDa bands appear to be diagnostic for natural infection.

DNA provides an excellent template on which to base a diagnostic assay, due to its stability and unique structure. Generic technologies exist for extracting nucleic acids from all classes of pathogens in a variety of different sample types, including tissues and blood. This extracted DNA can then be subjected to a number of assays that use a combination of base-pairing characteristics and DNA repair enzymes from hyperthermophilic bacteria to generate a diagnostic signal.

The DNA sequence of a gene characterized from three different, closely related organisms is shown (34). It can be seen that sequences consist of areas where the nucleotides are the same between the three species, whereas at other positions the bases vary. These sequence patterns reflect the fact that the product of the gene (e.g. an enzyme in this case) has areas that are critical and which must be composed of specific amino acids if the enzyme is to function and the organism to survive. Other positions, however, act as scaffolding to maintain the critical regions in the correct spatial orientation. In these areas the DNA and resultant amino acid sequence may be more variable. The degree of sequence conservation therefore varies between different regions of the same molecule. As two organisms evolve from a common ancestor, the nucleotide sequence of the genomes of the two progeny lines will change in a characteristic way. Mutations in non-critical regions of the genome are likely to be passed on to progeny and thus maintained, whereas the chance of a mutation in a critical region leading to a viable offspring, and thus transmission of this mutation, is much lower. This continuum of point mutation frequency allows discrimination between closely related organisms (which will differ in fast-changing non-critical regions) and more disparate organisms, where rare changes in critical regions will have occurred over a much longer time span.

All the methods described below exploit the fact that related organisms share DNA sequences; the more closely related two organisms are, the more highly conserved the nucleotide sequence of their genomes will be.

Probe-based hybridization assays

DNA is a very robust molecule. Its double helical structure can be 'unzipped' by heating or alkali treatment, without damaging the bonds between adjacent nucleotides. This results in two single-stranded molecules that can be immobilized (to stop re-annealing) onto inert supports such as nitrocellulose. These single-stranded molecules can then act as targets for labelled oligonucleotide probes, which are designed to have sequences complementary to a portion of the genome of a particular group of organisms (34). This is the basis for a variety of probe-based blotting/hybridization assays derived from the original method devised by Southern in the 1970s.

Originally, radioactively labelled probes were used and autoradiography was necessary to demonstrate that binding of probe to target had occurred. More recently, enzyme-linked probes have been developed that allow for chromogenic or chemiluminescent detection of binding events. Fluorescent dyes have also been used to allow visualization of probe binding.

34

```
Species A   1 5'ggttaacgat gttaacatga acgagtactg gtaccatttg aaaccagaca acggccagta 60
Species B   1 5'ggttaacgat gttaacatga tgcgattatc ctggataatg tcgagagtcg tgggcctcaa 60
Species C   1 5'ggttaacgat gttaacatga atgcgtacta gtaccattca attacacacc acggccagta 60


Species A  61 ggatcggttc gggttaccaa cttaaggcct gcccggcacg acactaattc ccgggtttaa3' 120
Species B  61 cgttgcgtag cggtgaccga tgtaagccga gcccggattg acactaattc ccgggtttaa3' 120
Species C  61 ccatcggtac tggttaccaa ttaaagggct gcccggatcg acactaattc ccgggtttaa3' 120
```

34 Sample DNA sequences of a hypothetical gene from three related organisms. If probes or primers complementary to the sequences in blue were produced, they would selectively hybridize to their parent organism's DNA but not with that of the two other organisms shown (providing the correct stringency conditions were used during the hybridization process). By contrast, probes designed to be complementary to either of the two longer conserved sequences (red) would bind to all three species.

In situ hybridization of probes (35) to bacterial or viral DNA is an excellent method for detecting low-grade infections in tissue sections or cytological preparations. As with most DNA-based methods, the equipment, expertise and time required limit their use as routine laboratory diagnostic tools or in-practice tests.

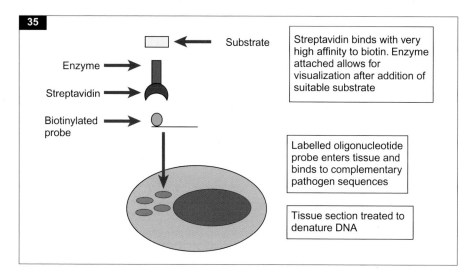

35 *In situ* hybridization. Enzyme-labelled oligonucleotide probes can be used to detect the presence of complementary DNA sequences in tissue samples. In this case a biotinylated oligonucleotide is shown.

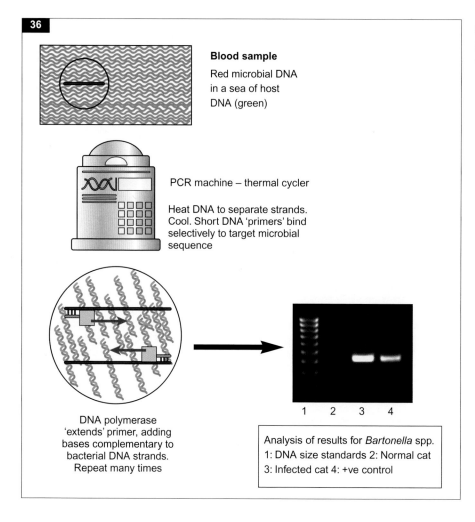

36 The polymerase chain reaction process as a diagnostic tool.

Polymerase chain reaction

Polymerase chain reaction (PCR) is a method that involves the amplification of target DNA sequences by repeated cycles of synthetic oligonucleotide primer-driven DNA synthesis. The key to the process is the use of a thermostable DNA polymerase (such as that derived from the hot spring bacterium *Thermus aquaticus*) that remains active after numerous cycles of heating to 94°C (201.2°F). Newly synthesized double-stranded DNA can thus be dissociated to act as templates for subsequent rounds of primer binding and DNA synthesis (**36**).

As the technology involved in determining the nucleotide sequences of pathogen genes has developed, a vast array of sequence information has been placed in databases such as GenBank. This information can be used to determine areas of genes that are conserved between species, genera and families of pathogenic organisms, or areas that are specific to individual strains. In parallel with this explosion of information, the commercial synthesis of oligonucleotide probes and the generation of economically priced, rapid DNA extraction kits mean that DNA-based diagnostic methods have become widely available. In many cases, where microbial culture is impossible, slow or undesirable due to biohazard considerations, PCR is becoming the method of choice in the diagnostic laboratory because of its sensitivity, selectivity and speed.

A recent development has been the linkage of fluorimetry and PCR in the process known as 'real-time' PCR. In this method, fluorescent dyes incorporated into reporter oligonucleotide probes, or dyes that bind to double-stranded DNA, are included in the reaction mixture (**37**, **38**). A number of different test formats are available but the common factor is that as PCR product is

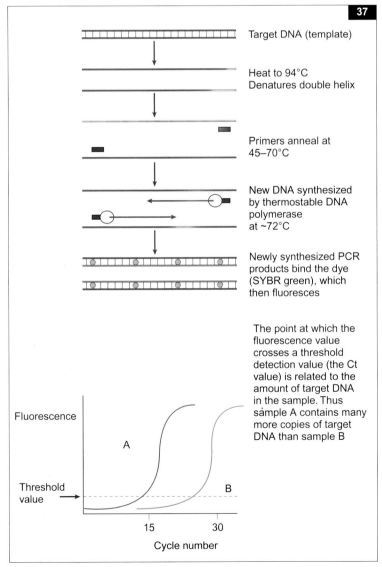

37

Target DNA (template)

Heat to 94°C
Denatures double helix

Primers anneal at
45–70°C

New DNA synthesized
by thermostable DNA
polymerase
at ~72°C

Newly synthesized PCR
products bind the dye
(SYBR green), which
then fluoresces

The point at which the fluorescence value crosses a threshold detection value (the Ct value) is related to the amount of target DNA in the sample. Thus sample A contains many more copies of target DNA than sample B

Fluorescence

A

Threshold
value

B

15   30

Cycle number

37 Real-time PCR using SYBR green.

38

Alternative method 1: 'Taqman' probes. An oligonucleotide with a fluorophore (F) at one end and a quencher (Q) at the other is called a Taqman probe. This binds to the middle of the amplified portion of template DNA. As the DNA polymerase copies the template it degrades the probe (P) releasing the fluorophore

Alternative method 2: Molecular beacons. A hybridization probe is designed that has a cental portion, which is complementary to the desired target. Each end of the probe has nucleotide sequences which are complementary to each other and allow base pairing to occur. The ends of the probe are labelled with a fluorescent reporter dye (R) and a quencher (Q). When the probe is 'zipped up' (no target template) there is no fluorescence but when template is available the probe unzips and fluoresces

38 Real-time PCR using alternative methods to generate a fluorescence signal.

produced the amount of fluorescence increases proportionately. Fluorescence is monitored throughout the assay and these data are converted into quantitative results reflecting the amount of pathogen in the sample (rather than the qualitative results given by conventional PCR). Therefore, this method has great advantages in assessing pathogen 'load' and responses to treatment.

The availability of machines that can monitor fluorescence at a number of different wavelengths has led to the development of multiplex assays where a number of different organisms, or gene targets, can be probed simultaneously. In multiplex systems, labelled probes are used, each of which has a reporter dye with a distinct, non-overlapping spectral signature. At each cycle during the assay, the machine assesses the fluorescence produced by the binding of each probe independently. This gives great savings in time, speed and cost of analyses, and the added bonus of absolute quantitation of each analyte.

The major problem with all PCR-based methodologies is their extreme sensitivity. This makes contamination a major concern, and laboratory design should consider the need to keep reagent preparation, DNA extraction from samples, thermal cycling and agarose electrophoresis analysis (where conventional PCR is used) physically separate to minimize the generation of false-positive results.

5 | Filarial infections

Luca Ferasin and David Knight

INTRODUCTION

Filarial infections (filariasis) are caused by roundworms (Phylum Nematoda) belonging to the ordor Spirurida, superfamily Filarioidea (commonly referred to as 'filarids'). There are approximately 200 species of filarial nematodes and some of them can cause severe pathologies in people and animals (*Table 6*). These parasites require an arthropod intermediate host, commonly a biting insect, to complete their biological cycle and for transmission. The first larval stages (L1) of these filarial nematodes are known as microfilariae and are found in the blood stream or in the subcutaneous tissues of the definitive host, from which they may be ingested during arthropod feeding. Adult nematodes may be found in a variety of different organs and tissues, depending on the species of parasite and the type of host. The microfilariae of each species have a characteristic morphology that may be used to diagnose the type of infection.

The primary pathological lesions occurring during filarial infections are caused by the presence of adults in a specific organ or tissue. However, the immune response against the parasites may also play a pivotal role in the pathophysiological mechanisms and, in many circumstances, microfilariae can also cause significant lesions.

Filarial infections are often classified according to the localization of the parasite within the host and the consequent pathological manifestations:

- Lymphatic filariasis (e.g. *Wucheria bancrofti* and *Brugia* species) is caused by the presence of nematodes in the lymphatic vessels.
- Subcutaneous filariasis (e.g. *Dirofilaria repens, Onchocerca volvulus, Loa loa, Dracunculus medinensis*) is caused by the presence of adults in the subcutaneous tissues, which can sometimes be seen migrating through the body.

Table 6 Biology and epidemiology of the principal agents of filarial infections.

Species	*Dirofilaria immitis*	*Dirofilaria (Nochtiella) repens*	*Dipetalonema reconditum*	*Brugia* species
Family	Onchocercidae	Onchocercidae	Setariidae	Onchocercidae
Common name(s) of the disease	Heartworm	Subcutaneous filariasis	Subcutaneous filariasis	Brugian filariasis, elephantiasis
Definitive hosts	Dogs, cats, wild canids and felids, sea lions, ferrets, humans	Dogs, cats, foxes, bears, humans	Canids	Humans, felids, dogs, monkeys
Intermediate hosts	Mosquitoes	Mosquitoes	Fleas, ticks, lice	Mosquitoes
Geographical distribution	Tropical, subtropical and warm temperate areas of the world	Southern Europe, Africa, Asia, USA, Canada	USA, Africa, Italy, Spain	India, Malaysia, South-east Asia
Morphology (adults)	m: 120–160 mm f: 250–300 mm	m: 50–70 mm f: 130–170 mm	m: 13 mm f: 23 mm	m: 20 mm × 200–300 μm f: 50 mm × 200–300 μm
Morphology (microfilariae)	300 × 8–10 μm	360 × 12 μm	270 × 4.5 μm	210 × 6 μm
Site of lesions (adults)	Right ventricle and pulmonary arteries; ectopic sites like eye, CNS, systemic arteries, body cavities	Subcutaneous tissues	Connective tissue; ectopic sites like body cavities and kidney	Lymph nodes and lymphatic vessels
Site of lesions (microfilariae)	Peripheral blood vessels	Peripheral blood vessels	Peripheral blood vessels	Lymphatic and capillary vessels

m = male; f = female

- Serous cavity filariasis (e.g. *Setaria* species, *Mansonella* species) is characterized by the presence of parasites in the pleural or peritoneal cavity.
- Cardiopulmonary filariasis (*Dirofilaria immitis*) is infection of the pulmonary arteries and the right side of the heart.
- Arterial filariasis (*Elaeophora schneideri*) is caused by the presence of adult worms in the systemic arteries.
- Ectopic filariasis is characterized by the incidental localization of a parasite in organs or tissues that are not typical of that particular species (e.g. presence of *D. immitis* in systemic arteries).

The biology and epidemiology of the filarial parasites affecting dogs and cats are shown in *Table 6*. The most important and geographically widespread filarial disease in the dog and cat is caused by *D. immitis* and is known as heartworm disease. *D. (Nochtiella) repens* is also frequently observed in pet animals and represents a more common zoonotic risk than *D. immitis*. *Dipetalonema reconditum* is another filarial nematode commonly found in dogs but with very little clinical significance.

Brugiasis (*B. malayi* and *B. pahangi*) is a filarial infection that affects lymph nodes and lymphatic vessels of dogs and cats in confined regions of south-east Asia.

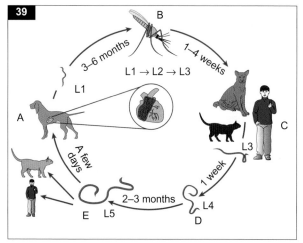

39 Life cycle of *Dirofilaria immitis*. (A) Adult worms in the pulmonary arteries and right ventricle of the definitive host release immature larvae (L1 or microfilariae) into the circulation. Microfilaraemia is uncommon in cats and humans. (B) Microfilariae are ingested by a mosquito during a blood meal and they mature from L1 to L3 in the insect. (C) L3 larvae penetrate the local connective tissues of the host during a later blood meal. (D) The larvae moult from L3 to L4. (E) L4 mature in the subcutaneous tissues until they reach the pre-adult stage (L5). L5 larvae migrate to the right heart and pulmonary arteries where they mature and mate, releasing microfilariae into the circulation and perpetuating the life cycle.

CARDIOPULMONARY DIROFILARIASIS (HEARTWORM DISEASE)

Background, aetiology and epidemiology

Dirofilariasis, or heartworm disease (HWD), is a filarial infection caused by *Dirofilaria immitis*. The parasite is primarily located in the pulmonary arteries and right heart of dogs and, less commonly, cats and ferrets. The infection can also occur in other species, such as wild canids, California sea lions, harbour seals, wild felids and humans, but these species are normally considered 'aberrant' or 'dead-end' hosts since the parasites rarely undergo final maturation to complete their biological cycle. *D. immitis* has also been described in horses, beavers, bears, raccoons, wolverines, muskrats and red pandas.

Life cycle

Dirofilariasis is transmitted by a mosquito bite (**39**) and there are more than 70 mosquito species that can potentially transmit the infection (see *Appendix*, p. 143).

Female *D. immitis* adults are viviparous and can release immature larvae (L1 or microfilariae) into the circulation. Microfilariae are ingested by a mosquito during a blood meal. Mosquitoes are not only vectors but also obligatory intermediate hosts and infection cannot be transmitted without a sufficient period of larval maturation (from L1 to L3) in the Malpighian tubules of the insect. The maturation period is variable, depending on environmental temperature. Development cannot occur below a threshold temperature of 14°C (57.2°F) and the cycle will be temporarily suspended until warmer conditions resume. When the average daily temperature is 30°C (86°F) the maturation can be completed in eight days, while it takes approximately one month when the environmental temperature is 18°C (64.4°F). As a consequence, transmission of infective larvae is limited to warm months and it varies depending on the geographical location.

The infective L3 larvae migrate from the Malpighian tubules to the lumen of the labial sheath in the vector's mouth and, during a later blood meal on an appropriate host, the L3 will exit the labium, enter the bite wound and penetrate local connective tissues. After approximately one week the larvae moult from L3 to L4 and, after a migration of 2–3 months in the subcutaneous tissues, moult to immature adults (L5). The L5 larvae penetrate a systemic vein and migrate to the right heart and pulmonary arteries within a few days, where they mature and mate after approximately 3–6 months, releasing microfilariae into the circulation and perpetuating their life cycle.

The life expectancy of *D. immitis* is approximately five years in dogs and two years in cats. In experimental infections the adult worms in cats do not reach the same size as in dogs, and their development is slower; therefore, the average prepatent period is longer in cats (eight months) than in dogs (5–6 months). Furthermore, the worm burden in cats is typically lower than in dogs and microfilaraemia is uncommon (less than 20% of infested cats) and, when present, it is inconstant and transient. Thus, cats are poor reservoirs of infection, as *D. immitis* is less likely to mature in this species and adults are short-lived when present.

Dirofilariasis is present in several countries, with a variable prevalence that depends on the canine population, the presence of mosquito vectors and the climate. The climate must be sufficiently warm to allow the presence of mosquitoes and the development of larval stages in the insects. For this reason, the prevalence of dirofilariasis varies with both geographical area and season. This is an important concept to consider when screening for the disease or planning a chemoprophylactic schedule.

The disease has been diagnosed throughout North America, in most countries of southern Europe and in Africa, Asia and Australia. In non-endemic countries, dirofilariasis may be diagnosed in dogs that have travelled from or through countries where infection is prevalent. However, at present, despite the presence of potential vectors and infected dogs, spread of disease is limited because of low average daily temperatures that do not support larval maturation within the mosquito. Climate change may result in the spread of infection into these areas in the future.

Pathogenesis

Dirofilariasis is primarily a cardiopulmonary disease. The presence of adult nematodes in the pulmonary arteries causes proliferation of the intima with consequent narrowing and occlusion of the vessels (**40–42**). Direct blockage by the adult worms is a less likely possibility. The severity and extent of lesions depend on the number and location of adult worms. The caudal lobar arteries are usually the most heavily parasitized. Severe pulmonary arterial disease may cause an increased permeability of lung vessels, with periarterial oedema and interstitial and alveolar cellular infiltrate, which can result in irreversible pulmonary fibrosis. Pulmonary thrombo-embolism (PTE) is another sequela of dirofilariasis. It is initiated as a consequence of platelet aggregation following exposure of collagen secondary to endothelial damage induced by the parasite (**40–42**). Platelet aggregation may also be responsible for the release of platelet-derived growth factor (PDGF), which promotes proliferation of medial smooth muscle cells and fibroblasts. PTE can also occur in response to adult worm death either as a spontaneous event or induced by adulticidal treatment. Experimental intravenous adminis-tration of *D. immitis* extract induces shock in dogs as a consequence of mast-cell degranulation and histamine release. This phenomenon seems to be caused by an unknown substance contained in the extract and may explain the circulatory collapse that is occasionally seen in dogs after the spontaneous death of parasites or adulticidal treatment.

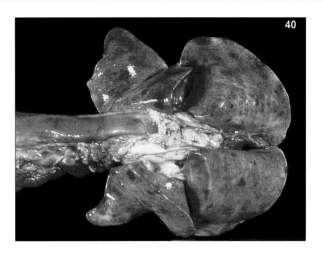

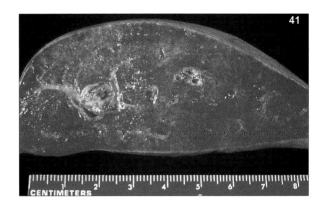

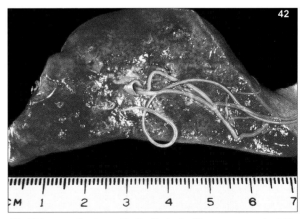

40–42 Lungs of a dog with dirofilariasis. The presence of adult nematodes in the pulmonary arteries causes proliferation of the intima, with consequent narrowing and occlusion of the vessels. Severe pulmonary arterial disease may cause increased permeability of lung vessels, with periarterial oedema and interstitial and alveolar cellular infiltrate. (**40**) The entire lungs appear oedematous, with areas of haemorrhagic infarction. (**41**) Section of a lung lobe showing inflammatory oedema and a large area of infarction. (**42**) Adult parasites in the lumen of a large pulmonary artery.

In cases of severe infection, particularly where a large number of parasites mature concurrently, retrograde migration from the pulmonary artery to the right ventricle, right atrium and venae cavae may occur (**43–45**). This induces incompetence of the tricuspid valve, which, in association with the concurrent pulmonary hypertension, is the cause of backward, right-sided heart failure (jugular distension, liver congestion, ascites) (**46**). Additionally, in heavy burdens, erythrocyte membranes may be damaged as cells pass through the mass of intravascular parasites, causing haemolysis and haemoglobinaemia. The presence of tricuspid incompetence,

right-sided heart failure with hepatomegaly, poor cardiac output and intravascular haemolysis with resultant haemoglobinaemia and haemoglobinuria is referred to as 'caval syndrome'. Severe cases of caval syndrome can also be characterized by the presence of adult worms in the caudal vena cava and thromboembolic events accompanied by disseminated intravascular coagulation (DIC). The pathogenesis of caval syndrome is not fully understood, even though the retrograde migration of adult nematodes from the pulmonary arteries to the right ventricle, right atrium and venae cavae seems the most convincing explanation.

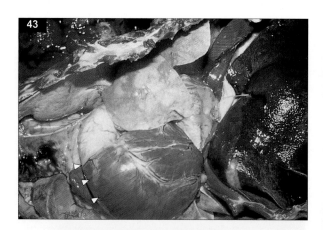

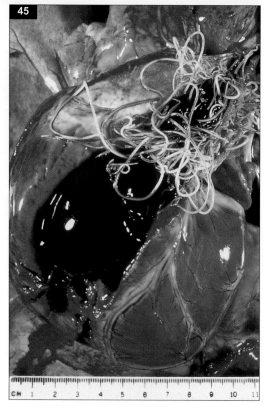

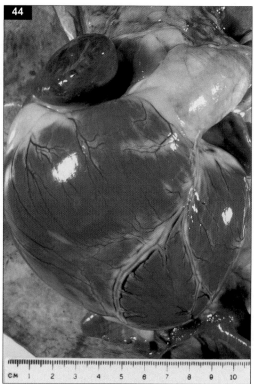

43–45 Necropsy specimens from a case of canine dirofilariasis. Right-side enlargement is primarily a consequence of the concomitant pulmonary hypertension. In cases of severe infection, migration of the parasites into the right ventricle and right atrium can contribute to the development of right heart enlargement. (**43**) Severe right ventricular enlargement (arrowheads). Hepatomegaly and liver congestion may also be appreciated. (**44**) Magnification of the same heart. The right side appears significantly larger than the left and there is gross dilation of the pulmonary artery. (**45**) Section of the right ventricle and pulmonary artery showing numerous adult parasites.

Immune-complex glomerular disease is also commonly reported in dogs with dirofilariasis. It is characterized by a protein losing nephropathy (PLN), with hypoalbuminaemia and, eventually, reduced plasma antithrombin III (ATIII), which may exacerbate the development of PTE. The antigen that causes the immune-complex disease is unknown but it could be a substance released by circulating microfilariae.

In cats, pulmonary hypertension, right-sided heart failure and caval syndrome are less common. In this species the presence of parasites in the distal pulmonary arteries may induce a diffuse pulmonary infiltrate and eosinophilic pneumonia. As in dogs, the subsequent death of adult parasites may cause acute pulmonary arterial infarction and the lung lobe involved can become haemorrhagic, with areas of oedema. If the cat survives the initial embolic lesion, recanalization around the obstruction occurs rapidly and pulmonary function can improve markedly within days, with remission of the clinical signs.

Occasionally, adult worms can migrate to sites other than the heart and the pulmonary arteries, and caused ectopic infection. Localization of *D. immitis* has been reported in the eye, CNS (cerebral arteries and lateral ventricles), systemic arteries and subcutaneous tissue. Ectopic infections are more commonly seen in cats than in dogs, suggesting that the parasite is not well adapted to feline hosts.

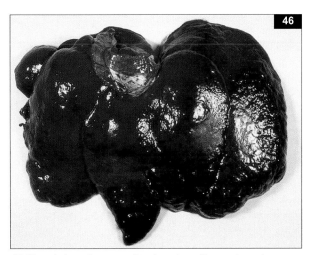

46 Chronic hepatic congestion in a dog with caval syndrome. Hepatomegaly is present and the parenchyma appears dark as a consequence of blood stasis. Eventually, the liver parenchyma may become fibrotic, with increased connective tissue and atrophy of the hepatocytes. These lesions are responsible for the portal hypertension and ascites.

Clinical signs

Dirofilariasis may be completely asymptomatic; however, clinical signs are generally present in cases with a high worm burden and/or when there is a significant allergic response of the host to the parasite. Infected patients may present with an acute onset of clinical signs but, more often, the disease develops slowly and gradually. Furthermore, clinical signs of dirofilariasis are triggered or exacerbated by exertion, and patients that perform little exercise may never show overt signs of HWD. In dogs, coughing is the most common clinical sign, followed by tachypnoea and dyspnoea, exercise intolerance, chronic weight loss and syncope. In severe cases, haemoptisis can be present as a possible consequence of pulmonary arterial rupture. Jugular distension, hepatomegaly, ascites and marked exercise intolerance are typical signs of right-sided heart failure. In these cases a systolic heart murmur or split second heart sound can be heard on thoracic auscultation, with a point of maximum intensity over the right apex. Hindlimb lameness and paresis have been described in dogs with aberrant arterial localization of the parasites.

Although the majority of infected cats are asymptomatic, cases of sudden death without any premonitory clinical signs have been described. Sometimes, sudden death is preceded by an acute respiratory crisis, probably as a consequence of filarial embolism and obstruction of a major artery. When present, clinical signs of dirofilariasis in cats are generally vague and non-specific. These may include anorexia, lethargy, coughing, vomiting, dyspnoea and collapse. In some cases the respiratory signs are very similar to those observed in cases of feline asthma.

Caval syndrome, a severe complication of HWD, is characterized by anorexia and weight loss, respiratory distress, haemoglobinuria secondary to intravascular haemolysis, signs of right-sided heart failure and possibly DIC.

Diagnosis

All diagnostic investigations are justified only if there is a previous history of exposure to mosquitoes in an area where *D. immitis* infection is likely to be present.

Laboratory diagnosis

A routine laboratory work-up is usually insufficient to make an aetiological diagnosis. Haematology often reveals eosinophilia and basophilia in the early stage of infection. Microfilariae can occasionally be seen on examination of the blood smear. Serum biochemistry may show changes related to secondary organ involvement (e.g. increased hepatic enzymes or increased blood urea and creatinine in cases of hepatic or renal damage respectively).

Cytological techniques

Cytology of bronchoalveolar lavage specimens may reveal the presence of numerous eosinophils 4–7 months after infection, especially in cats. However, differential diagnosis from feline asthma is often difficult.

Imaging

Survey radiographs of the thorax may show characteristic lesions, including main pulmonary artery bulge, enlarged and tortuous pulmonary arteries, and interstitial and/or alveolar pattern, especially in the caudal lung fields (**47, 48**). Moreover enlarged right ventricle and right atrium, enlarged caudal vena cava, hepatomegaly and ascites can be observed in caval syndrome. In cats the vascular changes are less frequently observed. They more commonly show radiographic changes similar to those observed in cases of feline asthma or *Aelurostrongylus abstrusus* infection, including overinflation of the lung accompanied by a broncho-interstitial, bronchial or alveolar pattern. Cats that have suffered recent episodes of pulmonary thromboembolism may show localized areas of increased lung opacity.

Non-selective angiography may help in the diagnosis of heartworm disease but it is rarely used because of the risks related to this procedure.

Adult heartworms can be visualized on echo-cardiography at the level of the main pulmonary artery, right ventricle and right atrium. They appear as a double-lined hyperechoic structure resulting from the echogenicity of the body wall of the parasite. A careful examination of the right parasternal short-axis basilar view at the level of emergence of the main pulmonary artery is especially recommended in cats in which the antigen test is negative but dirofilariasis is still suspected based on compatible clinical signs, radiographic changes and/or positive antibody test results. In cases of severe infection, echocardiography may also show right ventricular dilation and hypertrophy and Doppler study may confirm the presence of pulmonary hypertension and tricuspid insufficiency. Ultrasonography can also be particularly useful for the identification of parasites in ectopic locations.

Specific laboratory testing
Tests to identify microfilaria

A direct microscopic examination can be performed by depositing a drop of fresh blood under a cover slip. The motility of microfilariae creates turbulence of the surrounding red blood cells that can be easily observed under the microscope at ×100 magnification. This is a quick, easy and inexpensive procedure but lacks both sensitivity and specificity, particularly when low parasite burdens are present. The modified Knott's technique (centrifugation and staining with methylene blue) and filtration methods are more sensitive than direct microscopic examination and allow morphological examination of the microfilariae for species identification (**49**). In cats, given the absence or short presence of circulating L1 larvae, these tests have very little utility.

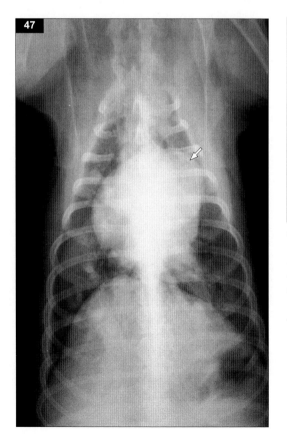

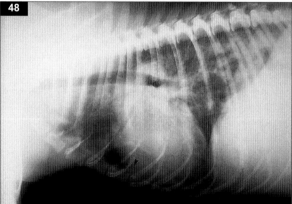

47, 48 Thoracic radiographs of a dog with dirofilariasis. (**47**) Dorsoventral view. The emergence of the main pulmonary artery is characterized by a prominent bulge (arrow). The right ventricle and right atrium are also enlarged. (**48**) Right lateral view. Enlarged and tortuous pulmonary arteries, and a mixed interstitial/alveolar pattern mainly affecting the caudal lung fields, are present.

49 L1 larva (microfilaria) identified by the Knott's test. The larva is surrounded by red blood cells and its dark colour is due to the methylene blue staining (×100 magnification).

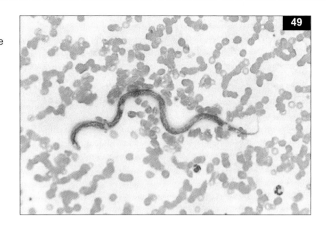

Antigen testing for dirofilariasis

The serological tests available for detecting heartworm antigens are summarized in *Table 7*. ELISA antigen tests detect specific circulating proteins released by the reproductive tract of the mature female worm, and a strongly positive antigen test is normally correlated with a heavy heartworm infestation. However, antigen level can also vary between animals with identical worm burdens. These tests are available either as 'in-clinic' tests or laboratory tests, and their sensitivity approaches 98% but decreases to 35% in dogs with low worm burdens. The antigen levels become undetectable 8–12 weeks after adulticidal therapy and this should be taken into account when re-screening for heartworm disease or evaluating the response to treatment. Specificity approaches 100% for all the available kits. Small worm burdens, the presence of immature females or male-only infections are common causes of low antigen titres and false-negative results, particularly in cats, where these circumstances occur more frequently. In dogs, specific immuno-chromatography techniques are also available. Antigen tests should be carried out at least seven months post infection in order to allow a sufficient concentration of antigens to accrue in circulating blood.

Table 7 Serological tests available to detect heartworm antigens in dogs and cats.

Test kit	Manufacturer	Type	Sensitivity (%) (Mean [range])	Specificity (%) (Mean [range])	Species	Type of sample
PetChek	IDEXX	ELISA	76 (66–98)	97 (90–99)	Dogs	S, P
SNAP canine HW	IDEXX	ELISA	67 (53–98)	98 (92–100)	Dogs	S, P, WB
SNAP feline HW	IDEXX	ELISA	73 (49–91)	99 (98–100)	Cats	S, P, WB
SoloStep CH	Heska	I-C	60 (44–97)	98 (92–100)	Dogs	S, P
Abboscreen	Abbott Lab.	I-C	52 (35–94)	96 (89–99)	Dogs	S, P
DiroChek	Synbiotics	ELISA	71 (59–98)	94 (86–97)	Dogs	S, P
DiroChek	Synbiotics	ELISA	79 (54–94)	98 (96–99)	Cats	S, P
Witness	Synbiotics	I-C	71 (69–92)	94	Dogs	S, P, WB

ELISA = enzyme-linked immunosorbent assay; I-C = lateral flow immunosorbent assay; S = serum; P = plasma; WB = whole blood; NA = published data not available.

Antibody testing for dirofilariasis

Antibody tests are currently available for routine screening of feline heartworm infection, either as 'in-clinic tests' or laboratory tests. They are summarized in *Table 8*. Antibody testing provides information about previous exposure but not necessarily about current infection. Consequently, antibody tests are more useful to rule out rather than confirm the infection. These tests are no longer used in dogs, given their low specificity and the widespread availability of highly reliable antigen tests.

PCR testing for dirofilariasis

PCR may represent a very sensitive and specific diagnostic tool for routine identification of mature and immature adult worms, especially in unconventional hosts. However, at present, this test is not widely available.

Treatment
Adulticidal treatment

The severity of the heartworm infestation should be carefully evaluated to determine the optimum treatment

Table 8 Serological tests available to detect heartworm antibodies in cats.

Test kit	Manufacturer	Type	Sensitivity (%) Mean (range)	Specificity (%) Mean (range)	Type of sample
SoloStep FH (5' incubation)	Heska	ELISA	32 (13–57)	99 (97–100)	S, P, WB
SoloStep FH (10' incubation)	Heska	ELISA	47 (24–71)	94 (91–97)	S, P, WB
SoloStep FH (20' incubation)	Heska	ELISA	84 (60–97)	85 (81–89)	S, P, WB
Assure FH	Synbiotics	ELISA	68 (43–87)	93 (89–95)	S, P
Witness	Synbiotics	I-C	NA	NA	S, P, WB

ELISA = enzyme-linked immunosorbent assay; I-C = lateral flow immunosorbent assay; S = serum; P = plasma; WB = whole blood; NA = published data not available.

Table 9 Classification of severity of heartworm infection in dogs.

	Class 1	Class 2	Class 3
Grade of severity	Mild	Moderate	Severe
Clinical complaints	None or occasional cough	Occasional cough, mild exercise intolerance	Persistent cough (± haemoptysis), moderate or severe exercise intolerance, weight loss, enlarged abdomen
Physical findings	Unremarkable	Mildly increased lung sounds	Abnormal auscultatory findings (split S2, gallop sounds, heart murmur, increased lung sounds); tachypnoea/dyspnoea, ascites
Radiographic changes	Unremarkable	Mild enlargement of pulmonary arteries, patchy alveolar/ interstitial infiltrates	Right heart enlargement, patchy or diffuse alveolar/interstitial patter, enlarged and tortuous pulmonary arteries, hepatomegaly, ascites
Echocardiographic changes	Unremarkable	Mildly enlarged pulmonary arteries and mild pulmonary hypertension	Severely enlarged pulmonary arteries and pulmonary hypertension, right ventricular and atrial enlargement
Prognosis	Excellent	Good in cases of successful treatment	Guarded

protocol and an accurate prognosis. A simple classification is available to assess the severity of the disease (*Table 9*). Dogs in class 1 carry a good-to-excellent prognosis after adulticidal therapy. However, if clinical signs are not apparent, immediate adulticide therapy may not be considered necessary and periodic clinical and radiographic monitoring could be a reasonable alternative. Dogs in class 2 may have a positive outcome but for those in class 3 the prognosis is guarded due to the high risk of therapy-induced parasitic thromboembolism. In the latter cases it is often difficult to decide whether adulticide treatment is warranted, and all the possible complications of adulticidal therapy should be thoroughly discussed with the owners.

In cats, adulticidal treatment can be dangerous even in patients with low-grade infection, and the risk of pulmonary thromboembolism due to premature parasite death is high. Some cats undergo spontaneous clinical remission after the natural death of *D. immitis* adults and, therefore, adulticidal treatment may not be warranted. Cats that show respiratory signs can be treated symptomatically as for feline asthma, with decreasing doses of prednisolone, starting at 2 mg/kg p/o daily and diminishing gradually until the lowest effective dose administered on an alternate daily basis is achieved. Cage rest, oxygen supplementation, fluid therapy, broncho-dilators and injectable steroids (e.g. dexamethasone) can be used to stabilize those cats that become acutely ill. Adulticidal treatment can be considered as the last resort for cats in a stable condition but with clinical signs that cannot be successfully controlled by the supportive therapy.

Melarsomine dihydrochloride is a new generation arsenical adulticide that is more expensive but offers several advantages over its predecessor thiacetarsamide. It is less nephrotoxic and hepatotoxic, requires only a two-dose protocol compared to the four required with thiacetarsamide, and has higher efficacy. Melarsomine is injected intramuscularly into the lumbar muscles at a recommended dose of 2.5 mg/kg and repeated after 24 hours. In order to reduce the post-adulticidal complications in class 3 dogs, only a single dose should be injected, followed one month later by the standard protocol of two injections 24 hours apart. This therapeutic strategy results in fewer worms being killed with the first injection and minimizes the risk of thromboembolism. Restricted exercise or cage rest, and corticosteroids at an anti-inflammatory dose, may help in minimizing PTE in the 7–10 days that follow the administration of melarsomine.

Sodium thiacetarsamide is an arsenical compound that has been used for decades in the treatment of HWD. The recommended treatment regimen is 2.2 mg/kg twice daily for two days by careful intravenous injection. However, production of thiacetarsamide has ceased and it is no longer available.

Macrolides
Macrolides are an alternative option when adulticidal treatment has been declined, as monthly administration of prophylactic doses will limit further infection. Furthermore, it has been shown that ivermectin and milbemycin may kill some adult nematodes.

Surgical removal of adult *D. immitis* in caval syndrome
Surgical heartworm removal has been well documented both in dogs and cats. Dogs with severe caval syndrome may benefit from the physical removal of worms from the right heart and pulmonary arteries with flexible crocodile or basket-type retrieval forceps. This procedure can reduce the risk of thromboembolism following adulticidal treatment and is also indicated for systemic arterial infections. The forceps technique requires general anaesthesia and fluoroscopic imaging. In dogs the expected outcome of this surgical procedure is positive in approximately 80% of cases. However, the anaesthetic risk, possible damage to cardiac structures and the potential hazard of postoperative ventricular arrhythmias should be carefully evaluated.

Microfilaricidal treatment
After recovery from adulticidal treatment (4–6 weeks), circulating microfilariae should be eliminated. There are no approved drugs for microfilaricidal treatment but a single administration of ivermectin (50 µg/kg p/o) or milbemycin oxime (500 µg/kg p/o) in dogs has been shown to be highly effective in eliminating the microfilariae from the circulation within a few hours. Moxidectin and selamectin are also known to be potent microfilaricides but, at present, there are still minimal data on the use of these drugs as microfilaricides. The sudden death of a large number of microfilariae can cause anaphylactoid reactions associated with vomiting, diarrhoea, ptyalism and circulatory collapse. These adverse effects can be limited by simultaneously administering corticosteroids (e.g. prednisolone 1–2 mg/kg p/o or i/m) with the microfilaricidal drug.

Prevention
Chemoprophylaxis is recommended for all pets living in endemic areas during the transmission period. In northern Italy, for example, where there is a high prevalence of HWD, mosquitoes are present only during the warm months and chemoprophylaxis is only recommended between May and October. Veterinarians should be aware of the seasonality of mosquitoes in their geographical regions in order to prescribe chemoprophylaxis at the appropriate time of year. It is strategically important to rule out the presence of the infection with adequate tests before starting the administration of chemoprophylactic drugs.

Macrolides represent the most common and efficient prophylactic drugs. There are, at present, four approved macrolides for prevention of HWD (*Table 10*). Ivermectin (6–12 µg/kg p/o) was the first approved drug, followed by milbemycin oxime (500–1,000 µg/kg p/o), moxidectin (3–6 µg/kg) and topical selamectin (6–12 mg/kg). The prophylactic efficacy of macrolides is due to their ability to kill tissue-migrating L4 larvae of *D. immitis* up to the sixth week of infection. Therefore, macrolides provide a high degree of protection when administered on a monthly basis. Although some degree of adulticide effect has been documented for macrolides at a prophylactic dose, patients that have missed one or more months of prophylaxis should be tested for heartworm infection after six months. This problem can now be avoided by use of an injectable sustained-release formulation of moxidectin. This product is not available in all countries but it can confer complete protection against infection after exposure for at least six months.

A chemoprophylactic schedule should be considered in non-endemic regions when pets are travelling to areas where dirofilariasis is prevalent. If pets reside in an endemic area for less than 30 days, a single administration of a prophylactic agent immediately after their return to the country of origin would be sufficient to guarantee protection. Conversely, if pets are resident in an endemic area for more than 30 days, administration of a prophylactic drug on a monthly basis after their departure is recommended.

High doses of ivermectin and milbemycin oxime have been shown to be potentially toxic in about one-third of collies but side-effects are not observed when administered at the recommended doses.

Daily administration of diethylcarbamazine citrate (DEC) was used for decades as a protocol for HWD prevention. However, its use is now limited as macrolides provide a more practical, reliable and safer alternative. There is minimal residual action and discontinuation for only 2–3 days may eliminate protection. DEC does not have an immediate larvicidal effect and it should be administered daily during and for two months after exposure to infective mosquitoes.

OTHER FILARIAL INFECTIONS

Subcutaneous dirofilariasis
Subcutaneous dirofilariasis is mainly caused by *D. (Nochtiella) repens*, which parasitizes domestic dogs in Europe (especially Italy, Spain, Greece, Yugoslavia and France), Africa and Asia, and bears in the USA and Canada. *D. repens* has also been reported in wild dogs, cats and foxes (*Table 6*, p. 51). Subcutaneous diro-filariasis is transmitted by different species of mosquito (genera *Aedes*, *Anopheles* and *Culex*) than those involved in *D. immitis* transmission. However, the biological cycle of *D. repens* is very similar to that of *D. immitis* except that adult *D. repens* worms reside in subcutaneous tissues. The clinical significance of adult *D. repens* worms

Table 10 Chemoprophylactic drugs available for heartworm prevention.

Trade name	Manufacturer	Active ingredient	Species	Recommended frequency of administration	Route of administration
Heartgard (Cardotek)	Merial	Ivermectin	Dogs, cats	Monthly	Oral (chewable tabs)
Heartgard Plus (Cardotek Plus)	Merial	Ivermectin (+ pyrantel)	Dogs	Monthly	Oral (chewable tabs)
Advantage Duo	Bayer	Ivermectin (+ imidacloprid)	Dogs	Monthly	Topical ('Spot-on')
Interceptor	Novartis	Milbemycin oxime	Dogs	Monthly	Oral (flavour tabs)
Sentinel (Program Plus)	Novartis	Milbemycin oxime (+ lufenuron)	Dogs	Monthly	Oral (flavour tabs)
Proheart (Guardian)	Fort Dodge	Moxidectin	Dogs	Monthly	Oral
Proheart 6 (Guardian 6)	Fort Dodge	Moxidectin microspheres	Dogs	Every 6 months	Injectable
Revolution (Stronghold)	Pfizer	Selamectin	Dogs, cats	Monthly	Topical ('Spot on')
Filaribits Plus	Pfizer	Diethylcarbamazine citrate (oxibendazole)	Dogs	Daily	Oral

in dogs and cats has not been clearly defined but nodular skin lesions and abscesses have often been described in association with infection. Furthermore, the parasite and its microfilariae appear to produce toxic substances and induce immunological reactions. Treatment is achieved by surgical removal of the parasites from skin lesions and the same prophylactic scheme used for *D. immitis* is also effective in preventing *D. repens* infections.

Dipetalonema reconditum infection

This nematode is commonly found in dogs in the USA, Africa, Italy, Spain and Australia. Unlike *D. immitis*, *Dipetalonema reconditum* infection is not limited to warm months because it is transmitted by fleas (*Ctenocephalides* species, *Pulex* species), ticks (*Rhipicephalus sanguineus*) and lice (*Linognathus* species) (*Table 6*, p. 51). The biological cycle of *D. reconditum* is very similar to that of *D. repens* and the adults live within the dog's subcutaneous tissues. Development of L3 larvae in the intermediate host takes 7–19 days and the mechanism of entry into the definitive host is not definitely known. It is possible that the infected flea is ingested by the dog while grooming and L3 larvae are released and then penetrate the mucous membranes of the mouth. The prepatent period of *D. reconditum* is approximately 60–70 days.

The clinical significance of *D. reconditum* is limited, although it may induce eosinophilia. It may also confuse the diagnosis of *D. immitis* infection if microscopic examination of a blood sample alone is used. The microfilariae of *D. reconditum* have a distinguishing cephalic hook and are smaller and narrower than *D. immitis* (*Table 6*, p. 51).

Histochemical differentiation of *D. immitis, D. repens* and *D. reconditum* microfilariae

D. reconditum and *D. repens* can cause false positives in tests for circulating *D. immitis* microfilariae but they can be differentiated with acid phosphatase staining. *D. immitis* microfilariae concentrate the dye in two regions, namely the excretory and anal pores, while *D. repens* shows an acid phosphatase reaction exclusively in the anal pore and *D. reconditum* stains evenly.

HUMAN DIROFILARIASIS

Although humans are considered incidental hosts, *D. immitis* and *D. repens* infections have been frequently reported in people and they represent an important zoonotic risk. The parasitic lesions are generally benign but they may be misdiagnosed as more severe disease and prompt unnecessary diagnostic and therapeutic procedures.

D. immitis can cause pulmonary dirofilariasis in humans. This is normally caused by a single nematode that rarely reaches sexual maturation and, after having entered the right ventricle, dies and causes embolization and small lung infarctions, which subsequently appear as solitary nodules on thoracic radiography. Microfilaraemia and extrapulmonary dirofilariasis have also been described but they represent rare events.

D. repens is commonly found in people in different body locations, including conjunctiva, eyelid, scrotum, inguinal area, breast, arms and limbs. Diagnosis of human dirofilariasis depends mainly on microscopic evaluation of the morphological characteristics of the nematode in histopathological specimens. Recently, a PCR-based assay has been validated to identify the different parasites in humans, animals and vectors. However, this technique is not suitable for formalin-fixed specimens and can only be used with fresh or alcohol-fixed material. This is an important limitation because tissue biopsies are normally fixed in 10% neutral buffered formalin.

Acknowledgement

Dr David H Knight passed away in July 2002, a few days after the final revision of this chapter. Dr Luca Ferasin would like to acknowledge Dr Knight's precious contribution, valuable advice and encouragement in reviewing the manuscript. Luca Ferasin would also like to dedicate this chapter to his friend David and their common passion for rowing and canoeing.

6 Babesiosis and cytauxzoonosis

Peter Irwin

BABESIOSIS

Background, aetiology and epidemiology

Babesiosis is caused by tick-borne intraerythrocytic protozoan parasites of the genus *Babesia* and is one of the most common infections of animals worldwide. Babesiosis (also referred to as piroplasmosis) occurs in domesticated dogs and cats, wild Canidae (wolves, foxes, jackals and dingoes) and wild Felidae (leopards, lions), and is gaining interest as an emerging zoonosis in humans. In dogs and cats, babesiosis was originally viewed as a tropical and subtropical disease but in recent times it has been recognized with increasing frequency in temperate regions of the world.

The classification of *Babesia* species places them in the phylum Apicomplexa, the order Piroplasmida and the family Babesiidae. The taxonomy of *Babesia* species has relied primarily on morphological characteristics of the intraerythrocytic parasites (merozoites and trophozoites) and other life cycle observations. However, the traditional methods of classification are gradually being replaced by molecular biological techniques, as morphological features by themselves are not sufficient for species differentiation. Molecular phylogenetic analysis has been useful not only for defining the relationships between individual *Babesia* species but also for further elucidating the association between *Babesia* and closely related parasites such as *Theileria* species and *Cytauxzoon* species. The erythrocytic stages of all three genera are similar, yet they are differentiated by the presence of distinct exoerythrocytic life cycle stages within the vertebrate host for *Theileria* and *Cytauxzoon* and by transovarial transmission, which is a feature of *Babesia*.

Babesia parasites of the dog

Babesia parasites have been grouped informally into 'small' *Babesia* and 'large' *Babesia* within their vertebrate hosts and both types are recognized in dogs. The larger piroplasm in dogs, *Babesia canis*, is recognized to represent at least three (sub) species: *Babesia canis canis*, *B. canis rossi* and *B. canis vogeli*, which are currently thought to be transmitted by different tick vectors (*Table 11*, p. 64). Intracellular forms are variable in number and shape and are readily observed by light microscopy due to their relatively large size (50). A fourth, genetically distinct, large *Babesia* parasite was recently discovered in the blood of a dog receiving chemotherapy in the eastern USA (*Table 11*, p. 64).

Until recently it was assumed that *Babesia gibsoni* was the only small piroplasm to exist in dogs (51). It was originally described from India early in the last century and is considered to be widespread and endemic

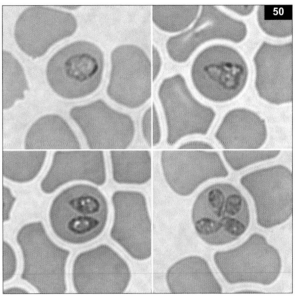

50 Large piroplasms of the dog (*Babesia canis vogeli*, northern Australia) demonstrating a variety of morphological forms.

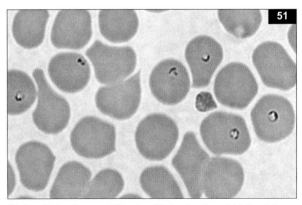

51 Small piroplasms of the dog (*Babesia gibsoni*, Malaysia). Note the small, single piroplasms in each erythrocyte. (Specimen courtesy of Dr EC Yeoh)

63

Table 11 Piroplasms affecting domestic dogs and cats, their tick vectors and a guide to their virulence.

Host	Type	Size (μm)	Piroplasm species (first description)	Distribution	Tick vector	Virulence
Dog	Large	2 × 5	*Babesia canis canis* (1895)	Southern Europe, Central Europe	*Dermacentor reticulatus*	Moderate/severe
			Babesia canis vogeli (1937)	Africa, Asia, N. and S. America, Australia, Europe	*Rhipicephalus sanguineus*	Mild/moderate
			Babesia canis rossi (1910)	Southern Africa	*Haemaphysalis leachi*	Severe
	Small	0.8–1.2 × 3.2	*Babesia gibsoni* (1910)	Asia, N. America, Australia, Europe	*Haemaphysalis longicornis*, *Haemaphysalis bispinosa*, *Rhipicephalus sanguineus*?	Moderate/severe
			Californian piroplasm (1991)	Southern California	Unknown	Moderate/ severe
			Spanish piroplasm = *Theileria annae* (2000)	Northern Spain	*Ixodes hexagonus*?	Moderate/ severe
		2.3 × 4	North Carolina piroplasm (2004)	North Carolina	Unknown	Uncertain (moderate: single isolate)
Cat		1 × 2.25–2.5	*Babesia felis* (1929)	Africa	Unknown	Mild/moderate
		1.7 × 2.7	Israeli piroplasm = *B. canis* subsp. *presentii* (2004)	Israel	Unknown	Uncertain (mild/moderate: 2 isolates)
		Unknown (DNA only detected)	*Babesia canis canis* (2003)	Spain, Portugal	Unknown	Uncertain (asymptomatic 3 isolates)
		1 × 2	*Cytauxzoon felis* (1979)	Southern States, USA, Zimbabwe	Unknown	Moderate/severe

throughout Asia. The full geographical range of *B. gibsoni*, as with the other canine piroplasms, has yet to be elucidated in detail but the organism has been found in dogs in the Middle East, parts of Africa, North America, Europe and most recently in Australia (*Table 11*). Reports of *B. gibsoni* from countries outside Asia are sporadic and probably reflect its introduction as a consequence of pets travelling across international boundaries.

A number of new canine piroplasms have been described and there is growing evidence that some of these should be classified as *Theileria* species rather than within the Babesiidae family (*Table 11*). It is likely that a better understanding of these species will be obtained as isolates from more locations around the world are investigated. A small piroplasm genetically distinct from *B. gibsoni* has been reported to occur in dogs in southern California (*Table 11*). This parasite has yet to be named but it is more pathogenic than the *B. gibsoni* infections reported in other regions of North America. Although morphologically similar to *B. gibsoni*, it displays a characteristic feature of 'Maltese cross' formation (a tetrad of parasites) within some red cells. It is also phylogenetically more closely related to piroplasms from humans and certain wildlife living in the western USA, which in turn possesses a close genetic relationship with *Theileria* species. A third small canine piroplasm has recently been found to be endemic in northern Spain (*Table 11*). This piroplasm (originally referred to as *Theileria annae*) closely aligns with *B. microti*, a parasite more commonly associated with rodent babesiosis.

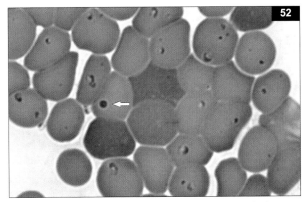

52 *Babesia felis* piroplasms in a cat with acute babesiosis (South Africa). Note the high parasitaemia and wide variety of morphological forms. There is also evidence of erythrocyte regeneration and the presence of single Howell Jolly body (arrow). (Specimen courtesy Dr T Schoeman)

Babesia parasites of the cat

Feline babesiosis appears to be less common and is not as well researched as the disease in dogs. The classification of *Babesia* in cats is far from clear at the present time and is based largely on morphological studies of parasites obtained from a variety of wild and domestic hosts. *Babesia felis* is currently recognized as the cause of babesiosis in domestic cats in parts of Africa (**52**). The association between the species found in wild (*B. herpailuri*, *B. cati*) and domesticated cats has yet to be determined and it is hoped that future studies using molecular tools will help to clarify the phylogenetic relationships of the feline *Babesia* parasites. Indeed, two new isolates recently discovered in the blood of cats in southwestern Europe and in Israel are most closely related to *B. canis* after gene sequence analysis (*Table 11*). Another closely related feline piroplasm, *Cytauxzoon felis*, is described later in this chapter.

Life cycle

Most *Babesia* parasites described to date are transmitted to their vertebrate hosts by the 'hard' ticks (Ixodidae). The life cycle of *Babesia* is summarized (**53**). Infective sporozoites are injected into the dog or cat within saliva during engorgement of the tick. These organisms then invade, feed and divide by binary fission within, and rupture erythrocytes during repeated phases of asexual

53 Life cycle of *Babesia* in the dog and invertebrate host (1) Sporozoites injected into bloodstream by feeding tick. (2) Trophozoite (ring form). (3) Merozoite. (4) Binary fission. (5) Paired trophozoites. (6) Infected erythrocytes ingested by feeding tick. (7) Lysis of erythrocyte in tick gut. (8) Gamont development and fusion. (9) Kinete formation. (10) Kinete migration from gut to other tissues within the tick, notably ovaries and salivary glands. (11) Development of sporokinetes in ovaries (ensuring transovarial transmission). (12) Development of sporokinetes to form a large, multinuclear sporont (containing many sporozoites). (13) Release of sporozoites from salivary gland during feeding. (Adapted from Melhorn H and Walldorf V (1988) Life cycles. In: *Parasitology in Focus: Facts and Fiction*. (ed. H Melhorn) Springer-Verlag, Berlin)

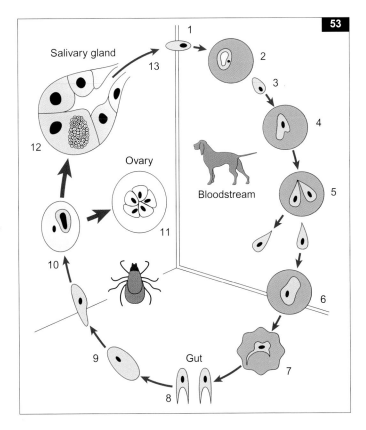

reproduction, releasing merozoites that find and invade other erythrocytes (54). In chronic infections it is assumed that babesial parasites become sequestered within the capillary networks of the spleen, liver and other organs, from where they are released periodically into circulation. Transmission to the vector may occur at any time that a parasitaemia exists. After ingestion by the tick, the complex processes of migration and sexual reproduction (gamogony and sporogony) take place, resulting in sporozoite formation in the cells of the tick's salivary glands. While tick transmission is the major source of infection, babesiosis may also occur after transfusion of infected blood and in neonates after transplacental transfer.

Epidemiology

In endemic regions the prevalence of antibodies directed against *Babesia* ranges from 3.8% to 80%, with the highest seroprevalence rates reported from animal refuges and greyhound kennels. A higher prevalence of babesiosis has been reported in male dogs and, generally, younger dogs (and cats) are more likely to develop clinical disease. The efficiency of tick control largely determines the risk of infection to individual household pets. A higher prevalence of *B. felis* infections has been observed in Siamese and Oriental cats in South Africa and there is an overrepresentation of Bull Terrier breeds in reports of *B. gibsoni* infections outside Asia, and in the Tosa breed in Japan. These latter associations have prompted the suggestion of horizontal (direct dog-to-dog) parasite transmission through biting, and the possibility of vertical (dam-to-pup) transmission in these breeds.

Babesiosis is considered to be an emerging disease in many parts of the world. Veterinarians should retain a high degree of clinical suspicion when faced with cases of haemolytic anaemia and should include questions relating to the pet's travel history during consultation. An increasing number of cases of canine babesiosis are reported in regions where the disease was not previously known to exist (e.g. northern Europe). Possible reasons for this include changing ecological and environmental

circumstances that favour the establishment of vector ticks in previously non-enzootic regions, and the increasing ease of international pet travel associated with the relaxation of national quarantine regulations. The brown dog tick *Rhipicephalus sanguineus* is particularly adaptable and may become established in homes with central heating, well beyond its usual enzootic range.

Concurrent infection with other haemoparasites, notably *Ehrlichia* species, *Mycoplasma* (*Haemobartonella*) species, *Hepatozoon* species and other species of *Babesia*, appears to be a common occurrence in endemic regions and potentially complicates the diagnosis and management of individuals by the veterinarian. Multiple co-infections are difficult to diagnose without highly sensitive tests such as PCR.

Pathogenesis

The severity of babesiosis in dogs and cats ranges from the development of mild anaemia to widespread organ failure and death. The critical determinant of this variable pathogenesis is the species or strain of *Babesia* parasite, yet other factors such as the age and immune status of the host and the presence of concurrent infections or illness are also important. While haemolytic anaemia is the principal mechanism contributing to the pathogenesis of babesiosis, it has been recognized for many years that the level of parasitaemia does not correlate well with the degree of anaemia, suggesting that multiple factors contribute to erythrocyte destruction. Direct parasite-induced red cell damage, increased osmotic fragility of infected cells, oxidative injury and secondary immune-mediated attack of the erythrocyte membrane result in a combination of intravascular and extravascular haemolysis.

The wide spectrum of clinical signs associated with canine babesiosis has led to the classification of uncomplicated and complicated forms.

Uncomplicated babesioisis

Uncomplicated babesiosis is generally associated with mild-to-moderate anaemia, lethargy, weakness and hepatosplenomegaly, and is typical of *B. canis vogeli* infections for example. Pyrexia, when it occurs, is attributed to the release of endogenous pyrogens and inflammatory mediators from inflamed and hypoxic tissue.

Complicated babesiosis

Complicated babesiosis refers to manifestations that cannot be explained as a consequence of a haemolytic crisis alone (*Table 12*). This form of babesiosis has been extensively studied in southern Africa, where it is associated with virulent *B. canis rossi* infection. Complicated babesiosis has been likened to human falciparum malaria and is characterized by severe anaemia and dysfunction of one or more organs. Cerebral babesiosis causes severe neurological dysfunction

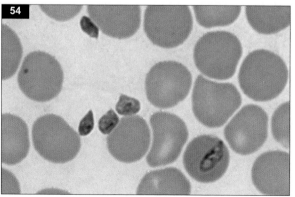

54 Free merozoites of *Babesia canis.*

Table 12 Features of complicated babesiosis.
• Anaemia (PCV < 0.15 l/l)
• Renal dysfunction
• Hepatic dysfunction
• Cerebral complications
• Rhabdomyolysis
• Pulmonary oedema
• Consumptive coagulopathy (DIC)
• Mixed acid-base disturbances

(seizures, stupor and coma) that is often peracute and associated with congestion, haemorrhage and sequestration of parasitized erythrocytes in cerebral capillaries. Hypotension and systemic inflammation are associated with the activation of cytokines and potent humoral agents such as kallikrein, complement and the coagulation systems. Consumption of platelets and clotting factors may result in haemorrhagic diatheses. Renal dysfunction has been attributed to the development of haemoglobinuric nephrosis but this probably requires additional processes such as hypoxia and reduced renal perfusion to become clinically evident (55, 56). A shift in haemoglobin-oxygen dissociation dynamics has been reported to occur in dogs with virulent babesiosis, leading to less efficient oxygen off-loading in capillaries, further compounding poor tissue oxygenation caused by the anaemia. Metabolic (lactic) acidosis in babesiosis has been attributed to anaemic hypoxia and capillary pooling. Recently, mixed respiratory and metabolic acid-base disturbances have been described in dogs with complicated babesiosis. With the buffering capacity of blood adversely compromised by low haemoglobin concentrations, arterial pH is reported to vary from severe acidaemia to alkalaemia. Mortality in complicated babesiosis often exceeds 80%.

Clinical signs
Canine babesiosis
Veterinarians should be mindful that the clinical picture of canine babesiosis might be complicated by concurrent infection with pathogens that share the same tick vector or result from sequential infections by different ticks. The most severe forms of the disease in adult dogs are generally associated with virulent infections (*B. canis rossi*, *B. canis canis*, *B. gibsoni* and the Californian piroplasm), yet pups are usually more severely affected than adults regardless of the babesial species. Ticks may or may not be found on the animal at the time of presentation in endemic regions but there is usually a history of known tick infestation or recent travel to a tick-enzootic region.

Peracute babesiosis, a feature of *B. canis rossi* infection, is characterized by the rapid onset of collapse. Clinical findings are typical of hypotensive shock and include pale mucous membranes (sometimes with cyanosis), rapid heart rate and weak pulse, profound weakness and mental depression. Fever may be present but hypothermia is a more consistent finding in this state. Severe intravascular haemolysis leads to haemoglobinuria ('red water'). This presentation is usually associated with complicated babesiosis, referred to in the previous section, and affected dogs develop signs that reflect widespread organ dysfunction associated with hypotension, hypoxaemia and extensive tissue damage such as anuria or oliguria, neurological dysfunction, coagulopathies and acute respiratory distress (*Table 12*). A rapid deterioration to coma and death is the usual outcome of peracute babesiosis.

Acute babesiosis is the clinical state that most veterinarians will encounter. Recurrent episodes may occur in some dogs infected with more virulent strains of the parasite (e.g. *B. canis canis*, *B. gibsoni*). Dogs with acute anaemia may have been unwell for a few days with non-specific signs such as anorexia, depression, vomiting

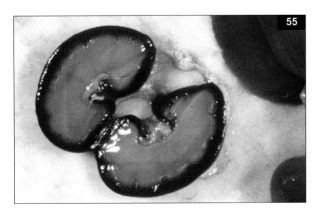

55 Sectioned kidney from a necropsy examination of a puppy that died of acute babesiosis, demonstrating the gross appearance of haemoglobinuric nephrosis in the renal cortex.

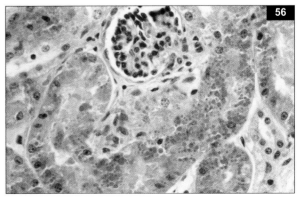

56 Haemoglobinuric nephrosis. High-power view of the renal cortex of the specimen in **55**, demonstrating hyaline droplet formation in the proximal tubules, confirmed to be haemoglobin by subsequent naphthol black staining.

and lethargy (57). The most consistent finding on physical examination is pallor of the mucous membranes, with a variable occurrence of fever, hepatosplenomegaly, icterus and dehydration (*Table 13*). Congested membranes are also occasionally reported. Petechial and ecchymotic

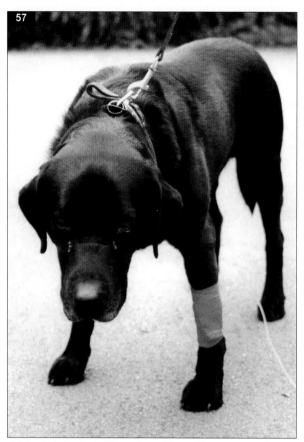

57 Acute babesiosis (*B. canis canis*) causing severe weakness and haemolytic anaemia in a six-year-old Labrador Retriever.

haemorrhages may be observed on the gums or ventral abdomen in some dogs, consistent with the presence of concurrent thrombocytopenia or thrombocytopathy. This may also suggest concomitant infection with a rickettsial organism. Urine obtained from dogs with acute *B. canis* infection is typically brown or dark yellow-orange, reflecting a mixture of haemoglobinuria and bilirubinuria. The patient's serum is often overtly haemolysed or icteric. A variety of atypical manifestations of severe babesiosis (e.g. dermal necrosis, myositis, polyarthritis) have been reported but the possibility of these being attributable to co-infection has not been examined in detail.

It is likely that most dogs that survive the initial infection become lifelong carriers of the parasite despite appropriate treatment and resolution of the original signs. Secondary immune-mediated complications such as anaemia, thrombocytopenia and glomerulonephritis may develop but in general the consequences of chronic infection are poorly understood. Many dogs remain subclinical, in a state referred to as premunity, despite intermittent, low parasitaemias. Recrudescence of intraerythrocytic parasites into the bloodstream may occur following stressful situations, immunosuppressive therapy or concurrent disease. In some individuals this leads to a further significant disease episode, yet others may develop only a mild anaemia and intermittent pyrexia. Chronic babesiosis has also been associated with non-specific signs such as anorexia, weight loss and lymphadenopathy. Although recurrent infections in the same dog may occur, in practice it is rarely possible to distinguish between recrudescence and a novel infection in endemic regions.

Feline babesiosis

South Africa appears to be the only country where feline babesiosis is currently recognized as a clinical entity in domestic cats; it tends to manifest as an afebrile, chronic, low-grade disease. Presentation of individuals to the

Table 13 Clinical features of babesiosis.

Uncomplicated		Complicated
Mild-to-moderate anaemia (PCV 0.15–0.35 l/l)	Severe anaemia (PCV <0.15 l/l)	Severe anaemia (PCV <0.15 l/l)
May be asymptomatic	Lethargy	Haemoglobinuria
Lethargy	Weakness	Oliguria or anuria
Fever	Fever	Shock-like state
Hepatosplenomegaly	Anorexia	Tachypnoea, dyspnoea, cough
Anorexia	Vomiting	Neurological signs (depression, collapse,
Pallor	Dehydration	seizures, vestibular signs, coma)
Mild icterus	Haemoglobinuria	Petechial and ecchymotic haemorrhage
	Icterus	Vomiting
Low mortality	Moderate mortality	High mortality

veterinarian may be delayed when compared with dogs, due in part to the more introverted nature of cats and to the failure of the owners to recognize early signs of illness. Furthermore, cats are able to tolerate more severe anaemia than dogs without showing signs. Anorexia, depression and pallor were the clinical signs attributed to feline babesiosis most commonly in one study, with weight loss, icterus, constipation and pica recorded less frequently. Pyrexia is not a feature of feline babesiosis. The highest prevalence of disease occurs in young adult cats (<3 years old) during the spring and summer in enzootic regions. Complications of feline babesiosis are wide ranging and include hepatopathy, renal failure, pulmonary oedema, cerebral signs and immune-mediated haemolytic anaemia. Concurrent infections with feline immunodeficiency virus, feline leukaemia virus and *Mycoplasma (Haemobartonella)* species may occur in older individuals. It is probable that young cats in enzootic areas contract the infection early in life and become subclinical carriers.

Diagnosis

The definitive diagnosis of babesiosis currently requires visualization of the parasite during light microscopic examination of a blood smear. It is expected that the application of new, highly sensitive molecular techniques such as PCR will complement the traditional methods of diagnosis in the future.

Identification of the *Babesia* species, or at least a distinction between 'small' and 'large' babesial organisms, is essential with regard to the choice of therapeutic agent. The search for *Babesia*-infected erythrocytes in a blood smear may be tedious and time-consuming when the parasitaemia is low, yet is greatly facilitated by the preparation of good quality blood films (*Table 5*, p. 42). Blood smears should be stained with a Romanowsky stain (such as May-Grünwald/Giemsa). Some of the rapid (Quick) stains that are available for in-house use are reported to result in inadequate parasite staining. The blood smear should be viewed through a cover slip, which is placed over the slide on a drop of microscope oil, or resin fixative (e.g. DPX) if a permanent mount is to be made. Large *Babesia* trophozoites can be seen using an objective lens magnification of ×40, but oil-immersion (×100 objective lens) is required for accurate identification of small babesial parasites. *Babesia* parasites should be differentiated from stain artefact and *Mycoplasma (Haemobartonella)* species by a magenta-staining nucleus and their blue and white cytoplasm (50, 51). In cats, *Cytauxzoon felis* appears very similar to *Babesia* species and accurate differentiation may require molecular techniques. Parasitaemias in cats with *B. felis* infection are variable and range from very low in chronic disease to extremely high in acute cases (52).

The physical properties of erythrocytes are altered after infection by *Babesia* parasites. Infected red cells become rigid, slowing down their passage through capillary networks. Large numbers of parasitized cells may be observed in capillary networks (58), a phenomenon that is possibly explained by the tendency of the parasite to proliferate locally in certain capillary beds or by the tendency of parasitized erythrocytes to autoagglutinate. This characteristic is useful for diagnosis as higher parasitaemias can be demonstrated in blood samples collected from the ear tip (59) and toenail.

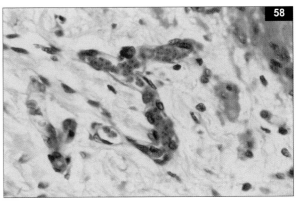

58 High-power view showing the accumulation of large numbers of parasitized erythrocytes within a capillary.

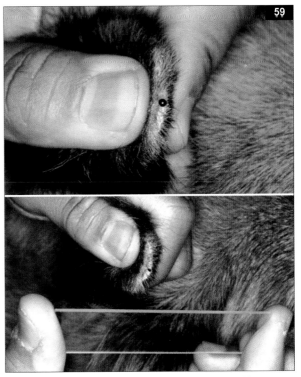

59 Preparation of an ear tip capillary smear. Fur should be removed from the tip of the pinna with scissors or electric clippers and the skin cleaned with a dry swab to remove skin squames and dirt. The ear tip should be gently pricked with a fine (25-gauge) needle and pressure applied to squeeze out a droplet of blood (**top**). A clean microscope slide is touched onto the drop of blood and a smear is made in the usual way (**bottom**).

Erythrocytes parasitized by the larger *Babesia* species are less dense than normal red cells and they concentrate in a layer immediately below the buffy coat within a haematocrit tube (**60, 61**). Parasitized erythrocytes are also found in greater numbers around the periphery of the blood film and in the 'feather' at the end of the smear.

Routine laboratory tests yield non-specific results in cases of babesiosis. Haematology typically reveals haemolytic anaemia, characterized by a regenerative anaemia, leucocytosis and thrombocytopenia. In peracute cases the anaemia is normochromic and normocytic, with erythron regeneration only evident after 2–3 days. Large 'reactive' lymphocytes (**62**) may be observed in chronic babesiosis, indicating antigenic stimulation, but they are also associated with other infectious disease states. Thrombocytopenia appears to be a very common finding in babesiosis, although its clinical significance is unclear. Platelet counts are rarely critical (<10 × 10⁹/l), typically within the range 20–90 × 10⁹/l, and overt signs of a bleeding diathesis (petechial and ecchymotic haemorrhages) are relatively unusual. Concurrent ehrlichiosis might further exacerbate the potential for bleeding by causing platelet dysfunction. Autoagglutination has been reported in babesiosis and up to 80% of dogs give a positive result in direct antiglobulin (Coombs) tests, making the search for parasites imperative in order to make the correct diagnosis. Immune-mediated haemolytic anaemia is the main differential diagnosis for babesiosis but other causes of haemolysis should be considered (*Table 14*).

Serum biochemistry results are non-specific in babesiosis. Extravascular red cell lysis results in elevated serum bilirubin in both dogs and cats. Acute hepatocellular injury leads to markedly elevated levels of ALT and AP in dogs, whereas AP and GGT are generally normal in cats with babesiosis. Azotaemia was recorded

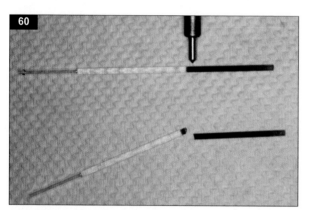

60 Erythrocytes containing large *Babesia* piroplasms accumulate just beneath the white cell layer (buffy coat) in a microhaematocrit tube. The tube should be cracked at this point with a diamond pencil to obtain a sample for a blood smear.

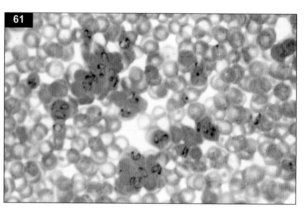

61 High-power view of concentrated parasitized erythrocytes obtained from beneath the buffy coat (see **60**).

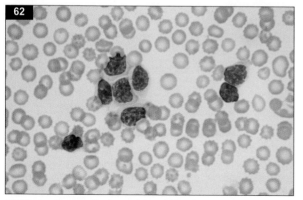

62 Photomicrograph of a peripheral blood smear demonstrating 'reactive' lymphocytes, which are a common feature of chronic babesiosis.

Table 14 Differential diagnosis of haemolytic anaemia in dogs.

Age of dog	Disorder
Neonates and young dogs	Neonatal isoerythrolysis
	Babesiosis
	Inherited erythrocyte defects (rare)
	Transfusion reactions
Older dogs	Immune-mediated haemolytic anaemia
	Babesiosis
	Heinz body anaemia (onion poisoning and various drug toxicities)
	Anticoagulant toxicity
	Dirofilariasis (caval syndrome)
	Transfusion reactions
	Acute zinc and copper toxicosis
	Neoplasia (microangiopathic haemolysis)

in 36% of dogs with Spanish piroplasm (T. *annae*) infection in northwest Spain and was associated with a high risk of mortality. Hyperkalaemia and hypoglycaemia have been reported in pups with acute intravascular haemolysis. Serum proteins are usually normal but hyperglobulinaemia with hypoalbuminaemia has been recorded in some chronic cases of babesiosis.

Because of the difficulty associated with the microscopic detection of babesial organisms, a variety of serological tests have been developed. These facilitate the identification of animals that have been exposed to *Babesia* parasites but provide little information about the individual's current infection status. The IFAT seems to be the most reliable assay for clinical purposes and is offered by commercial diagnostic laboratories in the USA and Europe. In this test, *Babesia*-infected erythrocytes are used as the antigenic substrate and positive reactions are detected indirectly in titrated serum samples by using an anti-canine globulin conjugated to a fluorescent marker. Specific methodologies vary between laboratories and the clinician should seek advice from the laboratory regarding accepted cut-off values. In most reports, titres exceeding 80 for *B. canis* and 320 for *B. gibsoni* are considered to be indicative of infection. Unfortunately, cross-reactivity between the canine babesial species often necessitates positive identification of the organism by microscopy. Antibodies to *Babesia* may also cross-react with *Neospora* or *Toxoplasma*, giving further potential for false-positive serology.

Amplification of *Babesia* DNA using PCR is a highly sensitive technique that is gaining wider acceptance as a diagnostic test, although it will be a few years before this type of testing becomes commercially available on a wider scale. Its particular value is likely to be for the detection of subclinical carriers in specific situations (e.g. before importation into *Babesia*-free regions) and for screening potential blood donors. Furthermore, real-time PCR may gain acceptance for quantitation of infectious load and for monitoring the effectiveness of therapy.

It is worth reiterating that the discovery of *Babesia* parasites in a blood film should always be viewed in the light of the clinical findings and other laboratory test results. It is not uncommon to find a low number of infected red cells in the blood of a clinically normal dog living in an endemic region.

Treatment

Issues to be considered when treating pets with a diagnosis of *Babesia* infection should include the clinical status of the patient, the degree of anaemia, the identity of the organism and its level of parasitaemia, and the potential for drug toxicity (especially if there is a history of previous anti-babesial therapy). In all but mild, uncomplicated cases, hospitalization and a combination of specific anti-babesial therapy and supportive care is necessary. Complicated babesiosis provides a challenge for even the most experienced intensive care clinicians. However, it is unrealistic to expect that specific treatment will sterilize

the babesial infection and, indeed, it may be preferable to induce a subclinical state of premunity in endemic regions where ongoing challenge is to be expected.

Specific therapy for babesiosis

Drugs that have been used for the treatment of babesiosis include the quinoline and acridine derivatives, the diamidine derivatives, the azo-naphthalene dyes, various anti-malarial formulations and assorted antibiotics, yet few have gained acceptance for being consistently reliable and safe. The choice of anti-babesial drug is determined largely by the species of *Babesia* infecting the patient, emphasizing the importance of an accurate recognition of the parasites during the diagnostic process. In general, imidocarb, diminazine, phenamidine, trypan blue and the combination of atovaquone and azithromycin are the preferred choices for canine babesiosis and primaquine is used for treating *B. felis* infections (*Table 15*, p. 72). Unfortunately, differences in national pharmaceutical registration laws mean that these drugs are not universally available.

Imidocarb

Imidocarb is an aromatic diamidine of the carbanilide series. In common with other diamidine derivatives, it interferes with parasite DNA metabolism and aerobic glycolysis, is rapidly effective and is slowly metabolized from the host. While it is generally safe for use in very young dogs with babesiosis, side-effects of imidocarb include pain at the site of injection and signs attributed to cholinergic properties of the drug, such as vomiting, diarrhoea, salivation, muscle tremor and restlessness (*Table 15*, overleaf).

Diminazine

Diminazine is a diamidine derivative used for the treatment of *B. gibsoni* infection, since imidocarb is less effective against the small babesial species. A single intramuscular dose is recommended for the treatment of canine babesiosis (*Table 15*, overleaf). The main disadvantage of diminazine is its low therapeutic index and, although the development of toxicity is dose-related in most dogs, there appears to be variable susceptibility between individuals and idiosyncratic reactions occur. Signs of toxicity can develop as soon as one hour after injection in some cases, or they may be delayed for up to 48 hours. Affected dogs show signs of central vestibular disease, including ataxia, rolling, vertical nystagmus and conscious proprioceptive deficits that may progress to opisthotonos, paralysis and death. Mild cases usually recover spontaneously but the worst affected dogs develop irreversible neurological deterioration. There is no antidote for diamidine poisoning so treatment should consist of supportive care. The toxicity of diminazine is cumulative and repeat injections should be avoided for at least 14 days. Diminazine has been successfully combined with imidocarb for treating *B. canis rossi* infections in South Africa, using a single injection of imidocarb

Table 15 Anti-babesial drug therapy.

Host	*Babesia* type	Drug name (and salt)	Recommended dose	Frequency	Notes/comments
Dog	Large	Imidocarb (dipropionate and dihydrochloride)	5 mg/kg s/c or i/m	Repeat after 14 days	Pain at site of injection and nodule may develop at site of injection. Cholinergic signs controlled with atropine (0.05 mg/kg s/c)
		Trypan blue	10 mg/kg i/v		Tissue irritant, use as 1% solution. Reversible staining of body tissues occurs
	Large and small	Phenamidine (isethionate)	15 mg/kg s/c	Once or repeat after 24 hours	Nausea, vomiting and CNS signs are common side-effects
		Pentamidine (isethionate)	16.5 mg/kg i/m	Repeat after 24 hours	
		Diminazine (aceturate and diaceturate)	3.5 mg/kg i/m	Once	Unpredictable toxicity, CNS signs may be severe. Some preparations contain antipyrone
	Small	Parvaquone	20 mg/kg s/c	Once	
		Atovaquone and	13.3 mg/kg p/o	q8h for 10 days	Atovaquone should be give with a fatty meal
		azithromycin	10 mg/kg p/o	q24h for 10 days	Atovaquone preparations containing proquanil cause side-effects
Cat	*B. felis*	Primaquine (phosphate)	0.5 mg/kg p/o	Once	

(6 mg/kg) followed by diminazine (3.5 mg/kg) the next day. This combination is apparently safe but consecutive injections using other diamidine derivatives, such as pentamidine or phenamidine, should be avoided on account of their cumulative toxicity. There have been additional concerns about the use of diminazine in severe, complicated babesiosis due to its hypotensive and anticholinergic effects. For such cases it is advisable to start intensive supportive therapy prior to administering the anti-babesial drug. Furthermore, some clinicians prefer to use another anti-babesial drug (e.g. trypan blue) initially in these cases. Diminazine is also safe for use in very young dogs with babesiosis but strict attention must be paid to the individual's body weight to avoid overdosing.

Atovaquone and azithromycin
A combination of the hydroxynaphthoquinone drug atovaquone and the macrolide antibiotic azithromycin is a welcome recent addition for the treatment of *B. gibsoni* infection (*Table 15*). The advantages of this drug combination are its safety (compared with diminazine) and the oral formulations, which permit medication by the owner at home. Although an optimal dose regime has yet to be determined, treatment with atovaquone and azithromycin results in a rapid reduction in parasitaemia but, as with other anti-babesial treatments, elimination of infection is not always achieved.

Other anti-babesial drugs
Trypan blue was one of the earliest drugs to be used for canine babesiosis but experience with this drug appears to be limited to South Africa. It is relatively safe and is thought to suppress parasite numbers by preventing their invasion of erythrocytes. Primaquine is an antimalarial that is considered to be the most effective drug against *B. felis* infection (*Table 15*). Although it reduces the parasitaemia (which can be extremely high in cats), it does not sterilize the infection. Accurate dosage calculations are required in cats in order to avoid toxicity; however, vomiting is a common side-effect at the recommended dose rate. Parvaquone may be used to treat

Table 16 Drugs used for supportive care of canine babesiosis.

Uncomplicated	Complicated
Blood transfusion (packed RBC or whole blood)	Blood transfusion (whole blood)
Crystalloid infusion if dehydrated	Crystalloid and colloid infusion as dictated
Dexamethasone? (0.2 mg/kg i/v once)	by patient's status
	Dexamethasone? (0.2 mg/kg i/v once)
Outpatient medication	**Pulmonary oedema**
Prednisolone?	Frusemide (2–4 mg/kg i/v or s/c q6–8h)
	Oxygen therapy
	Acute renal failure
	Frusemide (2–4 mg/kg i/v q6–8h)
	Mannitol 10% (1–2 g/kg i/v once) OR dopamine
	(1–5 µg/kg/minute i/v)
	Disseminated intravascular coagulation
	Plasma transfusion with heparin (75 units/kg
	added to plasma bag)
	Heparin (75 mg/kg s/c q8h)
	Outpatient medication
	Prednisolone?

small canine piroplasms (*Table 15*). This drug has proven efficacy against *Theileria* species and the close phylogenetic relationship of some of the canine piroplasms to these theilerial species may explain why parvaquone is effective. There is anecdotal information that doxycycline is effective against both large and small canine piroplasms but convincing evidence for this claim is currently unavailable.

Supportive care for babesiosis

Proactive supportive care is an integral component of the treatment of a dog or cat with babesiosis (*Table 16*). Regular patient monitoring should include assessment of mucous membrane colour, hydration status, respiratory rate and pattern and urine production, and laboratory evaluation of packed cell volume (PCV), serum total protein (TP), electrolytes and acid-base status. In dogs with severe anaemia, normalizing circulatory status is best accomplished by blood transfusion. Both the rapidity of onset and the degree of anaemia should be considered when assessing the need to provide additional red cells. Blood transfusion is generally indicated in dogs with a PCV of <0.20 l/l and cats with a PCV of <0.15 l/l. While in dogs it is preferable to confirm compatibility of the donor blood prior to transfusion by cross-matching, in cats this is mandatory due to the high prevalence of alloantibodies in this species. The development of 'in-house' blood-typing cards has greatly facilitated the assessment of donor-recipient blood compatibility in recent years (**63**). Fresh whole blood transfusions are preferred for complicated babesiosis cases but packed red cells are adequate in other cases (*Table 17*).

Table 17 Formulae for blood transfusion.

Whole blood transfusion:

Blood volume to be transfused

$$= k \times \text{body weight (kg)} \times \frac{(\text{required PCV} - \text{recipient PCV})}{\text{PCV of donated blood}}$$

Constant 'k' = 90 in dogs, 60 in cats

Packed red blood (pRBC) cell transfusion:
Infusion of 10 ml/kg pRBC will increase the recipient's PCV by approximately 10% (0.1 l/l)

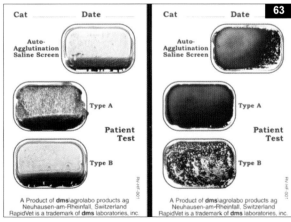

63 Cards for in-house determination of feline blood types. The presence of agglutination indicates the blood type. The sample on the left is type A and the sample on the right is type B.

Crystalline fluid therapy should be given with caution in anaemic patients in order to avoid causing further haemodilution or exacerbating respiratory distress. Oxygen therapy does not alleviate the hypoxia in anaemic states but is indicated for the therapy of pulmonary oedema in complicated babesiosis. Bicarbonate therapy continues to attract controversy and its use is best restricted to institutions where acid-base status can be regularly assessed and interpreted. Organ dysfunction associated with complicated babesiosis should be managed according to the general guidelines provided in current critical care manuals. A detailed review pertaining to the supportive treatment of canine babesiosis has been published (see Further reading, p. 146). Glucocorticoids, including dexamethasone and prednisolone (or prednisone), have been recommended by some authors but their benefits in babesiosis are currently unproven.

Prevention and control

As with any tick-transmitted disease, removing all possibility of exposure to the vector is the best way to prevent babesiosis. However, this is rarely achievable in endemic areas despite attentive ectoparasite control. Regular spraying, dipping or bathing with topical acaricidal preparations in accordance with the manufacturers' instructions should be practised in regions where tick challenge is continual. For dogs that are visiting tick-enzootic regions for a short time, and in cats that may have increased susceptibility to the toxicity of many acaricidal preparations, fipronil spray or 'spot-on' is a suitable choice, with a reasonable prophylactic effect. Owners should be encouraged to search their pets daily for ticks and, once found, to physically remove and dispose of them. Tick 'removers' have become available commercially in recent years and the use of these devices (and the wearing of gloves) may help to reduce the chance of inadvertent exposure of the owner to other potentially infectious agents within the tick (e.g. *Borrelia* species).

Several drugs have been investigated for their prophylactic potential against babesiosis, yet none have been consistently reliable in this regard. Experimental studies have suggested that a single dose of imidocarb dipropionate (6 mg/kg) protects dogs from *Babesia* challenge for up to eight weeks, and that doxycycline at 5 mg/kg/day ameliorates the severity of disease when challenged with virulent *B. canis*. Higher doses of both drugs may protect more effectively for longer periods but the potential toxicity of imidocarb and the overuse of doxycycline would be of concern. Reliance on such strategies cannot be recommended.

Vaccines made from cell culture-attenuated antigens have been developed for immunization against *B. canis canis* and are available commercially. While these vaccines do not prevent infection, they limit the parasitaemia and ameliorate the clinical signs and laboratory changes that occur after acute infection. The use of vaccines containing *B. canis canis* antigen only is restricted to Europe, as cross-protection against other *Babesia* parasites of dogs (e.g. *B. canis rossi* and *B. gibsoni*) does not develop. However, when mixed *B. canis canis* and *B. canis rossi* antigens are incorporated into a vaccine, heterologous protection is induced.

Zoonotic potential/public health significance

Babesiosis is an emerging zoonosis in many parts of the world yet, with a few exceptions, the babesial parasites of companion animals have not been implicated in zoonotic transmission. The majority of human cases of babesiosis in North America are associated with *B. microti*, a natural parasite of rodents, and these are typically mild or asymptomatic except in those individuals who are immunocompromised or splenectomized. In Europe, human babesiosis is less common but is associated with greater morbidity (and mortality) and is usually caused by the bovine pathogen *B. divergens*. In 1991 an acute malaria-like syndrome in a human patient on the west coast of the USA was attributed to a new *Babesia*-like piroplasm, designated WA-1. Molecular phylogenetic analysis has revealed that WA-1 is closely related to the small canine piroplasms (*Table 11*, p. 64) and falls within a cluster that includes *Theileria equi* (*B. equi*). A similar piroplasm, designated CA-1, was discovered in several splenectomized humans in California and is related to, yet distinct from, WA-1 and *B. gibsoni*. Serological surveys have been used to investigate the prevalence of babesial infections in regions where clinically apparent cases have occurred. Surveys of blood donors have shown 3–8% prevalence for *B. microti* and up to 16% prevalence of antibodies against the WA-1 organism.

CYTAUXZOONOSIS

Background, aetiology and epidemiology

Cytauxzoonosis is a tick-transmitted protozoal disease of clinical importance for domestic cats in southern regions of the USA. The causative agent is *Cytauxzoon felis*, which is recognized to have both pre-erythrocytic and erythrocytic phases of its life cycle in the vertebrate host. The exoerythrocytic stage of the life cycle has led to its taxonomic classification within the family Theileriidae, in the order Piroplasmida. Members of the genus *Cytauxzoon* are differentiated from *Theileria* species based on the fact that schizogony in *Cytauxzoon* occurs in macrophages, while schizogony in *Theileria* occurs in lymphocytes. However, it is clear that *C. felis* not only shares morphological characteristics with organisms of the genera *Theileria* and *Babesia* but it is also closely related on a molecular basis to the smaller piroplasms *B. rodhaini* and *T. equi* (formerly *Babesia equi*).

The natural hosts are the North American wildcat species such as the bobcat (*Lynx rufus*) and Florida panther (*Puma concolor coryi*) and it is thought that transmission of *C. felis* to domestic cats represents the inadvertent infection of a dead-end host. Natural *C. felis* infection may result from transmission by an attached tick, ingestion of infected ticks or by inoculation of

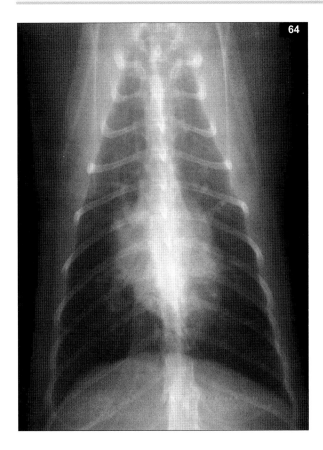

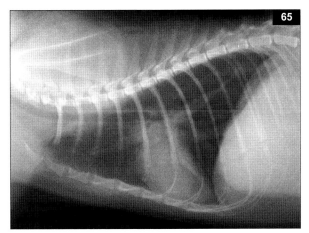

64, 65 Ventrodorsal (**64**) and lateral (**65**) radiographs of the thorax of a cat with cytauxzoonosis. The pulmonary vessels are enlarged and appear increased in number. The margins are slightly hazy due to a moderate diffuse increase in interstitial opacity, with a mild bronchial component. Faint pleural fissure lines indicate a small volume of pleural effusion. (Radiographs courtesy Dr N Lester).

infected blood or tissue during fights, notably with bobcats. The highest incidence of disease occurs during early summer through to autumn, corresponding to the time when ticks are most active. More than one individual in a multicat household may be affected and it is wise to check the other cats when the disease is first diagnosed.

The life cycle of *C. felis* is poorly understood. It is suspected that *Dermacentor variabilis* is the principal vector for natural transmission and is responsible for injecting infective sporozoites from its salivary glands into the mammalian host. Schizonts develop primarily within tissue histiocytes in many organs and go on to release merozoites, which invade monocytes and erythrocytes. In cats that survive initial infection, low-level erythrocytic parasitaemias can persist for many years.

Pathogenesis

Infection of domestic cats with the schizogenous stage typically results in a rapidly progressive systemic disease with a high mortality rate. In natural infections with *C. felis* there is an apparent variation in pathogenicity that may be associated with geographical location. In one recent report, 18 cats living in an area near the northern border of Arkansas and Oklahoma survived natural infection and developed chronic parasitaemia. The pathogenesis of cytauxzoonosis is attributed to the schizogenous phase that causes mechanical obstruction to blood flow through various organs, notably the lungs, and results in a shock-like state. Vascular occlusion and damage are further associated with the release of inflammatory mediators and development of DIC. Intravascular and extravascular haemolysis occur as a result of erythrocyte invasion by merozoites.

Clinical signs

The tissue schizont phase of infection with *C. felis* is responsible for the clinical signs. Soon after infection, affected cats develop non-specific signs such as anorexia, lymphadenopathy, fever and lethargy, but the course of the disease is usually rapid, with the onset of a severe clinical syndrome characterized by dehydration, pallor, dyspnoea, icterus, recumbency and death. Thoracic radiographs may reveal enlarged and tortuous pulmonary vessels as a result of vascular occlusion by the tissue stages (**64, 65**). Usually, by the time the cat is presented, it is severely ill. Most cats die within 9–15 days following infection by virulent strains, regardless of treatment.

Diagnosis

The diagnosis of cytauxzoonosis is made by the identification of erythrocytic piroplasms in blood smears stained with Wright's stain or Giemsa (**66**). There is no serological assay commercially available at the current time. Parasitaemias are typically low (1–4%), although in some acute infections as many as 25% of the red cells may be infected. *C. felis* is a small piroplasm (*Table 11*, p. 64) that must be differentiated from *Babesia felis*, which is very similar in size and appearance, by light microscopy; however, *B. felis* is confined geographically to southern Africa. *C. felis* appears in a number of morphological varieties including the signet-ring form, bipolar oval forms, tetrads and dark-staining 'dots', the latter of which may be mistaken for a more common and widespread parasite of cats, *Mycoplasma* (*Haemobartonella*) species, the cause of feline infectious anaemia. A unique, yet uncommon, finding in cytauxzoonosis is the appearance of tissue phase schizonts in blood smears and buffy coat preparations. However, these forms are best demonstrated in impression smears from bone marrow, spleen or lymph nodes, where they are typically numerous (**67**).

Haematology and serum biochemistry abnormalities are typical of haemolytic anaemia. Initially, the anaemia is normochromic and normocytic but it progresses to a strong regenerative response, characterized by the presence of nucleated red cells by the time of death. Moderate to severe leucopenia is typical and thrombocytopenia, sometimes profound, is commonly reported with or without DIC. Prolongation of clotting times (PT and APTT) has been recorded and has been used to support a diagnosis of disseminated intravascular coagulation (DIC), but concentrations of fibrin degradation products (FDP) are variable. The plasma appears icteric on the last day or two of life and is associated with a high serum concentration of bilirubin. Other clinicopathological changes that have been recorded in cases of cytauxzoonosis include hyperglycaemia, hypokalaemia, hypocholesterolaemia and elevations in serum ALT and AP; however, these changes may be minimal in acutely affected individuals that typically die before such abnormalities are recorded.

Necropsy findings in cats that have died of cytauxzoonosis include pallor and icterus of the tissues, petechial and ecchymotic haemorrhages on the serosal surfaces of organs, oedematous lymph nodes and lungs, and hepatosplenomegaly. The diagnosis may be confirmed by histological examination of the tissues. Large numbers of mononuclear phagocytes containing schizonts are visible in the veins of most organs, including the liver, lung, spleen, lymph nodes, kidneys and CNS.

Treatment and control

The diagnosis of cytauxzoonosis carries a grave prognosis, with high mortality rates despite treatment. Of the specific therapies that appear to help ameliorate the disease, imidocarb dipropionate and diminazine aceturate have shown most promise (*Table 18*). It is suggested that these drugs are used in cats at lower doses than those usually recommended in dogs for the treatment of babesiosis, and both may transiently worsen the clinical status of the recipient. Early administration of subcutaneous heparin, together with fluid therapy and blood transfusions, may also be beneficial in the management of DIC, but controlled studies are lacking.

Zoonotic potential/public health significance

There is currently no recognized zoonotic potential of *C. felis* infection.

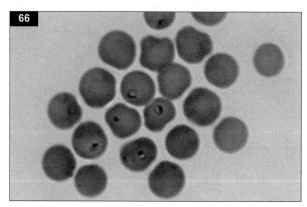

66 *Cytauxzoon felis* piroplasms in a domestic cat with terminal cytauxzoonosis (Oklahoma, USA). (Specimen courtesy Dr J Meinkoth)

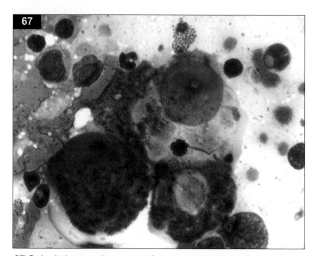

67 Splenic impression smear from a domestic cat that died from cytauxzoonosis. Note the large schizont-laden macrophages. (Specimen courtesy Dr J Meinkoth)

Table 18 Treatment of cats with cytauxzoonosis.

Type of therapy	Drug/medication	Recommended dose	Frequency	Notes/comments
Specific	Diminazine aceturate	2 mg/kg i/m	Once	Haemolysis and icterus may worsen transiently after injection
	Imidocarb dipropionate	2 mg/kg li/m	Repeat after 3–7 days	Anticholinergic signs (vomiting, diarrhoea, miosis, 3rd eyelid prolapse and muscle fasciculations) controlled by atropine (0.05 mg/kg s/c)
Supportive	Crystalloid fluid therapy	To correct dehydration and provide maintenance	Ongoing	Care to avoid excess haemodilution
	Blood transfusion	Refer to Table 17	As required	Blood typing or cross-match is necessary to ascertain compatibility of donor blood
	Heparin	100–150 units/kg s/c	q8h	Reduce dose gradually to avoid rebound hypercoagulability

Hepatozoonosis

Gad Baneth and Nancy Vincent-Johnson

CANINE HEPATOZOONOSIS

Background, aetiology and epidemiology

Canine hepatozoonosis is a tick-borne disease caused by apicomplexan protozoa from the family Hepatozoidae. Two distinct species of *Hepatozoon* are known to infect dogs: *Hepatozoon canis* and *Hepatozoon americanum*.

H. canis infection (HCI) was first reported from India in 1905 and has since been described in southern Europe, the Middle East, Africa, southeast Asia and South America (**68**). *H. canis* infects the haemolymphatic tissues and causes anaemia and lethargy. *H. americanum* infection (HAI) is an emerging disease in the USA that is spreading north and east from Texas, where it was originally detected in 1978. This organism infects primarily muscular tissues and induces severe myositis and lameness. *H. americanum* was initially considered a strain of *H. canis*, until it was described as a separate species in 1997. The species distinction was based on differences in the clinical disease manifestations, tissue tropism, pathological characteristics, parasite morphology and tick vectors. Subsequent genetic and antigenic comparative studies have supported the separate species classification (*Table 19*).

The main vector of *H. canis* is the brown dog tick *Rhipicephalus sanguineus,* which is found in warm and temperate regions all over the world. The Gulf Coast tick *Amblyomma maculatum* is the vector of *H. americanum*. *A. maculatum* exists in the southern part of North America, throughout Central America and in the northern part of South America. In the USA, *A. maculatum* was once confined to the warm, humid regions along the Gulf and South Atlantic coasts but recently its geographic range has expanded to reach as far inland as southern Kansas and Kentucky. Both of the *Hepatozoon* species that infect dogs are transmitted trans-stadially from the nymph to the adult stage in their tick vectors. Larval *A. maculatum* ticks can also become infected and transmit *H. americanum* as newly moulted nymphs or adults.

Whereas *H. canis* appears to be a parasite of canines that is well adapted to dogs, and causes only mild clinical signs in the majority of infections, it seems that *H. americanum* is less adapted to parasitic co-existence in the dog, causing a severe disease in most cases. It is possibly a parasite of some other animal in North America and is transmitted to dogs through ingestion of ticks that feed as nymphs or larvae on the natural host. Gamonts and meronts of a *Hepatozoon* species have been reported in coyotes, bobcats and ocelots in the USA. The majority of these animals were in good physical condition at the time of capture. *H. americanum* has been successfully transmitted to coyote puppies from *A. maculatum* ticks that had previously fed on infected dogs. In contrast to the infected adult animals, puppies developed clinical signs of myasthenia, pain, ocular discharge, leucocytosis and inappetence. They also developed bone lesions typically seen in dogs with HAI and one pup was infective to nymphal *A. maculatum* ticks.

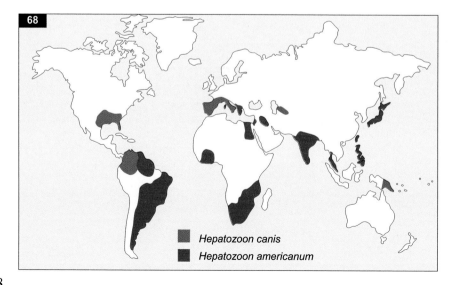

68 Reported geographical distributions of *H. canis* and *H. americanum*.

Table 19 Comparison of *Hepatozoon americanum* and *Hepatozoon canis* infections.

Organism	*H. americanum*	*H. canis*
Main clinical signs	Lameness Muscular hyperaesthesia Fluctuating fever Lethargy Mucopurulent ocular discharge	Fever Lethargy Emaciation
Severity of signs	Severe; signs may wax and wane	Often mild A severe disease is seen in dogs with a high parasitaemia
Haematological findings Extreme leucocytosis	Common, may be as high as $200 \times 10^9/l$	Rare, found in dogs with a high parasitaemia
Peripheral blood gamonts	Rare	Common
Parasitaemia	Usually < 0.1% of leucocytes	1–100% of neutrophils
Anaemia	Common	Common
Radiographic abnormalities	Periosteal proliferation of long bones	Non-specific
Main diagnostic method	Demonstration of cysts and pyogranulomas in muscle biopsy	Detection of gamonts in blood smears
Primary target tissues	Skeletal muscle, cardiac muscle	Spleen, bone marrow, lymph nodes
Histopathological abnormalities	Pyogranulomatous myositis	Splenitis, hepatitis, pneumonia
Distinct tissue parasitic forms	'Onion skin' cyst	'Wheel spoke' meront
Vector tick	*Amblyomma maculatum*	*Rhipicephalus sanguineus*
Therapy	Trimethoprim/sulphonamide Pyrimethamine Clindamycin Decoquinate	Imidocarb diproplonate Doxycyline

Life cycle and transmission

The life cycles of *H. canis* (**69**) and *H. americanum* (**70,** overleaf) include two hosts: the tick as a definitive host in which the sexual part of the cycle takes place, and a dog or other mammal as an intermediate host in which asexual reproduction of the parasite occurs. Nymphal or larval (in the case of *H. americanum*) ticks engorge with gamont-infected leucocytes while feeding blood on an infected intermediate host. Gamonts are freed from the leucocytes, associate in pairs in syzygy and transform into

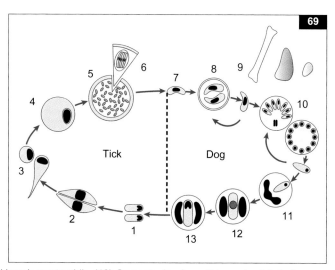

69 Stages in the life cycle of *H. canis*. (1) Gamonts ingested by a tick during a blood meal from a parasitaemic dog are released from neutrophils. (2) Gamonts associate in syzygy during gametogony. (3) Male and female gametes transform prior to fertilization. (4) A zygote develops into an early oocyst. (5) During sporogony, numerous sporocysts are formed within the oocysts. (6) Each sporocyst contains several elongated sporozoites. (7) After ingestion of an infected tick, sporozoites are released from the oocysts and penetrate the dog's intestinal tract. The sporozoites disseminate to target tissues, mainly haemolymphatic organs. (8) Meronts containing macromeronts are formed during merogony in the haemolymphatic tissues. (9) Merozoites release from ruptured mature meronts and repeat the cycle of merogony. (10) Elongated micromerozoites are formed within a 'wheel spoke'-type meront. (11) Micromerozoites free from mature meronts and invade neutrophils. (12) Gamonts develop within neutrophils in the haemolymphatic organs. (13) Neutrophils containing mature gamonts enter the blood circulation and are ingested by a tick on taking in a blood meal.

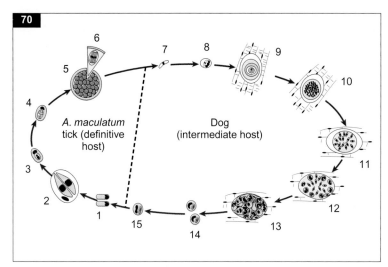

70 Stages in the life cycle of *H. americanum*. (1) Gamonts ingested by a tick during a blood meal from a parasitaemic dog are released from leucocytes. (2) Gamonts associate and undergo gametogony, after which fusion (syngamy) and fertilization take place within a tick gut cell. (3) Zygote development within a tick host cell. (4) Sporogony and formation of early sporocysts within the developing oocyst. (5) The mature oocyst contains over 200 sporocyts. (6) Each sporocyst contains 10–26 elongated sporozoites. (7) After ingestion of an infected tick, sporozoites are released from the oocysts and penetrate the dog's intestinal tract. (8) Sporozoites enter host cells and disseminate to target organs, mainly skeletal and cardiac muscle. (9) Layers of mucopolysaccharides are laid down around the parasite and host cell, forming an 'onion skin'-shaped cyst. (10) The parasite undergoes merogony within the cyst. (11) Mature merozoites are formed in the cyst. (12) Rupture of the cyst is followed by release of merozoites and induction of a local inflammatory response. (13) A pyogranuloma with intense vascularization is created where the cyst existed. Leucocytes are invaded by merozoites. (14) Some of the merozoites develop into gamonts, while others may disseminate to other muscular tissues and repeat merogony. (15) Mature gamonts in leucocytes enter the blood circulation and are ingested by a tick upon taking in a blood meal.

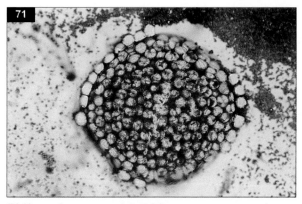

71 *H. americanum* oocyst containing numerous sporocysts.

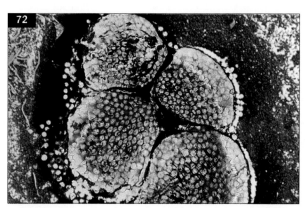

72 Four attached *H. americanum* oocysts in a haemocoele smear.

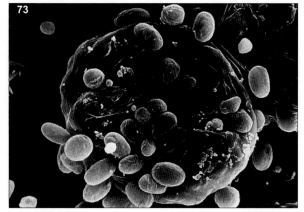

73 Scanning electron microscope image of an *H. canis* oocyst. The oocyst is enveloped by a membrane and surrounded by free sporocytes.

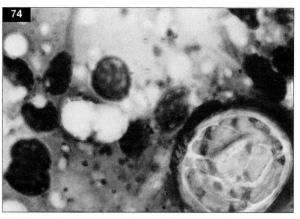

74 *H. americanum* sporocyst containing sporozoites.

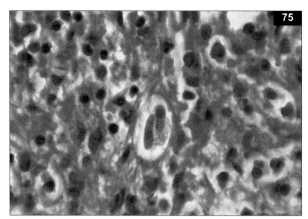

75 Two *H. canis* macromerozoites in a section of spleen from an experimentally infected dog.

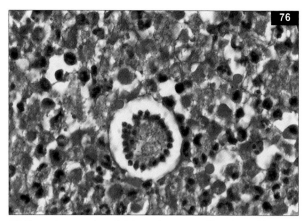

76 *H. canis* meront containing micromerozoites shaped in a 'wheel spoke' form in a section of spleen from a naturally infected dog.

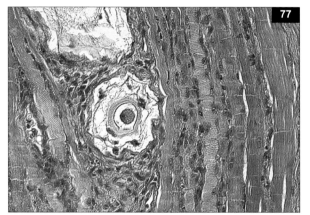

77 *H. americanum* cyst in skeletal muscle. Infrequently, the cyst is found with a developing or mature meront with merozoites.

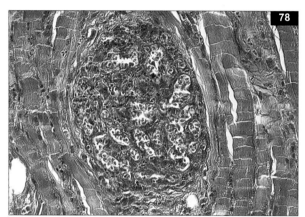

78 A pyogranuloma in muscle tissue from a dog with *H. americanum* infection.

male and female gametes. Fertilization occurs and results in the formation of zygotes that develop to oocysts. Each mature oocyst (**71–73**) contains numerous sporocysts (>200 for *H. americanum*) and 10–26 sporozoites develop within each sporocyst (**74**). After the tick moults, oocysts are found within the tick's haemocoele and each tick may carry thousands of infective sporozoites. *Hepatozoon* parasites have not been shown to migrate to tick salivary glands or mouthparts. Thus, transmission occurs by ingestion of an infected tick and not by a tick bite.

Once ingested by a dog or other susceptible mammal, the sporozoites of either species are released from the oocysts, penetrate the intestinal wall and are transported (possibly within a phagocytic cell) to target tissues and organs. *H. canis* disseminates via the blood or lymph and primarily infects the spleen, lymph nodes and bone marrow, where merogony takes place. Two forms of *H. canis* meronts are found in infected tissues: one type containing 2–4 macromerozoites (**75**) and a second type

containing more than 20 elongated micromerozoites (**76**). When the meront matures and ruptures, merozoites are released and penetrate neutrophils, in which they develop into gamonts that circulate in peripheral blood. *H. americanum* has an affinity for skeletal and cardiac muscle tissue, where it develops between myocytes within host cells of undetermined origin. Mucopolysaccharide layers encyst the host cell in the muscle (**77**), where the parasite subsequently undergoes merogony. At maturation the cyst ruptures, releasing merozoites into adjacent tissue. Neutrophils and macrophages are recruited to the area and may become infected, each with a single zoite. A pyogranuloma forms where the cyst once existed (**78**). Intense angiogenesis results in a highly vascular structure. It is hypothesized that this provides a route by which infected leucocytes re-enter the circulation either become circulating gamonts or distribute parasites to distant sites to repeat the asexual reproduction cycle. The life cycle of both *Hepatozoon* species is completed when ticks ingest blood infected with gamonts.

Experimental infections have shown that *H. canis* completes its development in the dog with the appearance of peripheral blood gamonts within 28 days post infection. *H. americanum* completes its life cycle in the dog within 32 days. The development of *H. americanum* in nymphal *A. maculatum* ticks from feeding to the observation of mature oocysts in the haemocoele of a newly moulted adult tick requires 42 days.

Other modes of transmission may exist. As with *Toxoplasma gondii*, some species of *Hepatozoon* can be transmitted through predation and ingestion of cysts present in tissues of intermediate hosts. This has not yet been documented for either *H. canis* or *H. americanum* but seems plausible. Vertical transmission of *H. canis* has also been reported in puppies born to an infected dam and raised in a tick-free environment. The importance of this mode of transmission in the epidemiology of the disease has not yet been determined.

Pathogenesis

Most dogs infected with *H. canis* appear to undergo a mild infection associated with a limited degree of inflammatory reaction. However, HCI may vary from being apparently asymptomatic in dogs with a low parasitaemia to life threatening in animals that present with a high parasitaemia. HCI can be influenced by immune suppression due to co-existing infectious agents, an immature immune system in young animals or the presence of a primary immunodeficiency. Immune suppression influences the pathogenesis of new *H. canis* infections or the reactivation of pre-existing ones. Treatment with an immunosuppressive dose of prednisolone is followed by the appearance of *H. canis* parasitaemia in dogs with experimental HCI. Concurrent HCI and infection with other canine pathogens are common; reported co-infections include parvovirus, *Ehrlichia canis*, *Anaplasma platys*, *Toxoplasma gondii* and *Leishmania infantum*.

In contrast, immunosuppression or concurrent illness is not necessary to induce clinical disease in dogs infected with *H. americanum*. The earliest lesions in skeletal muscle are noted three weeks post exposure, when the parasite may be seen within the host cell. Over time, the host cell produces the mucopolysaccharide lamellar membranes around itself to form the 'onion skin' cyst unique to *H. americanum* infection (**79**). Some cysts undergo merogony very rapidly while others appear to enter dormancy. Clinical signs in infected dogs result from the pyogranulomatous inflammatory response that occurs after the encysted mature meront ruptures, releasing merozoites into the surrounding tissue.

Prolonged infection may occur from a single infecting episode perpetuated by repeated merogonic cycles. Cysts of *H. americanum* may be found years after the initial diagnosis in clinically recovered dogs. It is likely that these cysts have the potential to reactivate, producing continued cycles of asexual reproduction. This may cause the waxing and waning pattern of clinical signs and relapse following treatment.

Clinical signs

Hepatozoon canis

Infection with *H. canis* may be subclinical in some animals but produce severe and fatal disease in others. It is difficult to characterize the clinical signs of HCI because: (1) dogs with low parasitaemia may be apparently asymptomatic; (2) the non-specific nature of changes such as pale mucous membranes due to anaemia, and lethargy; and (3) the involvement of concurrent diseases in some of the cases. Mild disease is common and is usually associated with low-level *H. canis* parasitaemia (1–5%), frequently in association with a concurrent disease. A more severe disease, characterized by lethargy, fever and severe weight loss, is found in dogs with high parasitaemia, often approaching 100% of circulating neutrophils (**80**). Dogs presenting with both leucocytosis and high parasitaemia may have a massive number of circulating gamonts (>50,000 gamonts/mm^3). This extensive parasitism takes its toll on the canine host by demanding nutrients and energy, by direct injury to the affected tissues and by activating the different branches of the immune system. This massive parasitic load may lead to extreme loss of weight and cachexia in dogs with a high parasitaemia, although the dogs sometimes maintain a good appetite.

Hepatozoon americanum

Dogs infected with *H. americanum* are often presented with gait abnormalities ranging from stiffness to complete recumbency, generalized pain and deterioration of body condition. On physical examination the most common findings include fever, pain or hyperaesthesia, muscle atrophy, weakness, depression, reluctance to rise and mucopurulent ocular discharge (**81**). Body temperature tends to correlate directly with waxing and waning of clinical signs and may range from normal to 41°C (106°F).

Hyperaesthesia and/or generalized pain result from both pyogranulomatous inflammation in skeletal muscle and the periosteal reaction that causes bony proliferation. Pain can manifest as cervical, back, joint or generalized pain and clinical signs may resemble those of meningitis or discospondylitis. Affected dogs may display a 'His Master's Voice' stance as a result of guarding the cervical region (**82**). Muscle atrophy becomes apparent with chronic disease and can result in secondary weakness. Most dogs maintain a relatively normal appetite throughout the course of the disease. Despite this, weight loss is common due to muscle atrophy and chronic cachexia. Mucopurulent ocular discharge is common and is sometimes associated with decreased tear production. It may coincide with fever spikes and owners often report that the ocular discharge is the first noticeable sign of clinical relapse. Transient diarrhoea, often bloody, has been reported. Less frequently reported clinical signs include polyuria and polydipsia, abnormal lung sounds or cough, pale mucous membranes and lymphadenomegaly.

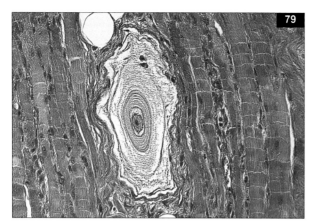

79 *H. americanum* cyst. The round-to-oval 'onion skin'-shaped cysts are 250–500 μm in diameter. The outer portion of the cyst is made up of concentric layers of fine, pale blue-staining laminar membranes. A developing parasite may sometimes be observed at the centre of the cyst.

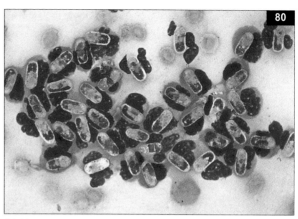

80 *H. canis* gamonts on the edge of a blood smear from a naturally infected dog with extreme leucocytosis and a high parasitaemia approaching 100% of the neutrophils.

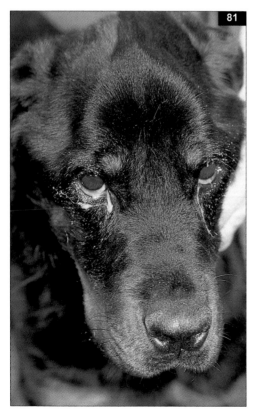

81 Rottweiler naturally infected with *H. americanum*, with typical mucopurulent ocular discharge and facial muscle atrophy.

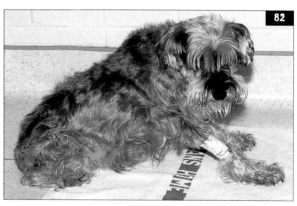

82 Miniature Schnauzer naturally infected with *H. americanum* exhibiting 'His Master's Voice' stance due to severe musculoskeletal pain and excessive stiffness.

Laboratory findings

Most dogs with HCI have white blood cell counts within the reference range. However, dogs with a high parasitaemia frequently have extreme neutrophilia (up to 150×10^9/l), although it is less common than in dogs with HAI. Normocytic, normochromic non-regenerative anaemia is the most common haematological abnormality reported in HCI. Less frequently, a regenerative anaemia, sometimes severe, may be seen. In a case-controlled study of dogs with *H. canis* parasitaemia admitted to a veterinary teaching hospital in Israel, dogs with hepatozoonosis were significantly more anaemic than the control hospital population admitted with other diseases, and dogs with high parasitaemia were more anaemic and had higher leucocyte counts than both the controls and the dogs with low parasitaemia. Thrombocytopenia and proteinuria have also been reported in HCI.

In dogs with HAI, the most outstanding haematological abnormality is marked leucocytosis, characterized by neutrophilia. The white blood cell count typically ranges from $20–200 \times 10^9$/l, with reported means of 76.8 and 85.7×10^9/l. A mild to moderate normocytic, normochromic, non-regenerative anaemia is typical. Thrombocytosis, with platelet counts of $422–916 \times 10^9$/l, occurs in a considerable number of dogs. Thrombocytopenia is rare unless there is concurrent infection with *Ehrlichia canis*, *Anaplasma platys*, *Rickettsia rickettsii* or other tick-borne organisms.

Abnormalities in serum biochemistry in highly parasitaemic dogs with HCI include hyperproteinaemia with hyperglobulinaemia and hypoalbuminaemia, and increased creatine kinase (CK) and alkaline phosphatase (AP) activities. In dogs with HAI the most common biochemical changes are a mild elevation in AP and decreased albumin. Artefactual hypoglycaemia (in the range of 2.22–3.33 mmol/l and occasionally as low as 0.28 mmol/l) due to increased *in vitro* metabolism by the elevated number of white blood cells may be seen if sodium fluoride is not used for sample collection. The low albumin has been attributed to decreased protein intake, chronic inflammation or renal loss. Blood urea nitrogen (BUN) is also frequently decreased below the reference range. Surprisingly, CK activity is typically normal despite the myositis caused by *H. americanum*. Although the decreases in albumin and BUN are suggestive of hepatic failure, both fasting and postprandial bile acids are usually within the reference range or only slightly elevated.

Radiographic findings

Dogs with HAI commonly develop osteoproliferative lesions. Periosteal new bone formation is typically disseminated and symmetric and is usually most frequent and severe on the diaphysis of the long bones. The radiographic appearance of the bony lesions ranges from subtle bone irregularity to a dramatic smooth laminar thickening (**83**). A study of the formation of the bone lesions after experimental infection with *H. americanum*

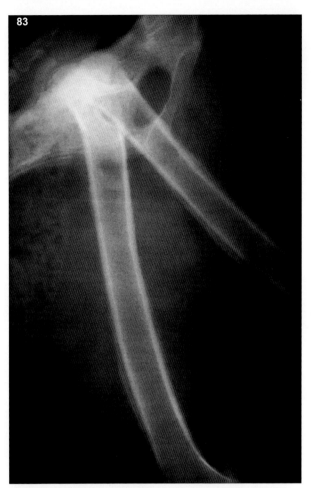

83 Radiograph showing periosteal proliferation of the femurs and pelvic bones in *H. americanum* infection. Bone lesions range from rough irregularity to smooth laminar thickening such as in this case.

revealed that the stages of morphologic development of the lesions very closely resemble those of hypertrophic osteopathy.

Diagnosis

HCI is usually diagnosed by microscopic detection of *H. canis* gamonts in the cytoplasm of neutrophils, and rarely monocytes, on Giemsa- or Wright's-stained blood smears. They have an ellipsoidal shape, are about 11×4 μm and are enveloped in a thick membrane (**84**). Between 0.5% and 5% of the neutrophils are commonly infected, although this may reach as high as 100% in heavy infections. A case-controlled study of dogs with *H. canis* parasitaemia admitted to a veterinary hospital in Israel indicated that 15% had a high number of circulating parasites (>800 gamonts/mm³).

In contrast to *H. canis*, gamonts are infrequently found on blood smears from dogs infected with *H. americanum*. When they are identified, it is usually in very low numbers, rarely exceeding 0.1% of the leucocytes examined (85). Gamonts may exit the leucocytes rapidly after blood is drawn, leaving behind an empty capsule that is difficult to identify. Consequently, blood smears should be made rapidly after sampling to enhance identification. Buffy coat smears will also increase the chance of gamont detection. Bone marrow aspirates usually show granulocytic hyperplasia with an increased myeloid:erythroid ratio, and lymph node aspirates often reveal lymphoid hyperplasia. However, neither procedure is useful in making a definitive diagnosis as organisms are rarely seen in these samples.

Radiography of the limbs or pelvis can be used for screening a suspected animal because many dogs with HAI will show periosteal proliferation. However, muscle biopsy is a more consistent method of diagnosis of HAI as it typically reveals the unique cyst and pyogranuloma formation associated with *H. americanum* (77–79).

Myositis with muscle atrophy, necrosis and infiltration of inflammatory cells between muscle fibres is a frequent finding. The parasites are widely distributed in the muscle tissue but multiple biopsies are recommended to increase the chances of detecting the organism, especially in early or low level infections. The biceps femoris, semi-tendinosus or epaxial muscles are recommended sites for biopsy.

An indirect fluorescent antibody test (IFAT) and western blot for the detection of anti-*H. canis* antibodies were developed using gamont antigens (86). The IFAT has been used for epidemiological studies in Israel and Japan. A survey of dogs from Israel showed that 33% had been exposed to the parasite as indicated by the presence of anti-*H. canis* antibodies. Only 3% of the seropositive dogs had detectable blood gamonts and only 1% had severe clinical signs associated with the infection. This indicates that although there is a wide exposure to

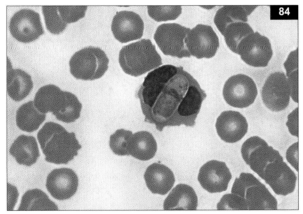

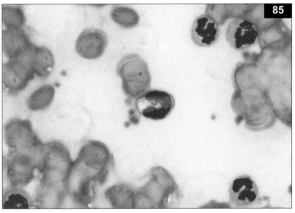

84 Single *H. canis* gamont on a blood smear from a naturally infected dog. Note the ellipsoidal shape of the gamont compressing the lobulated neutrophil nucleus towards the cell membrane.

85 Blood smear showing a gamont of *H. americanum* in a neutrophil. Although similar in appearance, the gamonts of *H. americanum* are slightly smaller in size than those of *H. canis* (8.8 × 3.9 µm compared to 11 × 4 µm).

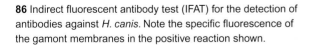

86 Indirect fluorescent antibody test (IFAT) for the detection of antibodies against *H. canis*. Note the specific fluorescence of the gamont membranes in the positive reaction shown.

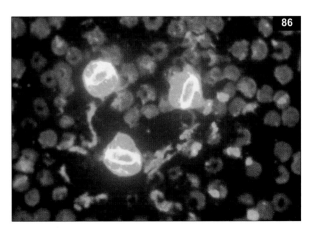

H. canis, most infections are probably subclinical. IgM and IgG class antibodies to *H. canis* were detected by IFAT in experimentally infected dogs as early as 16 and 22 days post infection, respectively, well in advance of gamont detection by microscopy at 28 days post infection. Antibodies detected by IFAT may be formed against conserved antigens found in earlier life cycle stages of *H. canis*.

Sera from dogs infected with *H. americanum* showed only a low degree of cross-reactivity to *H. canis* antigens by IFAT. However, an ELISA for *H. americanum*, using sporozoites as antigen, was reported to have a sensitivity of 93% and a specificity of 96% when compared with muscle biopsy.

Necropsy findings

HCI may be found as an incidental finding in histopathological specimens from dogs from endemic areas. In dogs with a low parasitaemia, few tissue lesions may be identified. However, necropsies of dogs with a high parasitaemia reveal hepatitis (87), pneumonia and glomerulonephritis associated with numerous *H. canis* meronts. Meronts and developing gamonts are also found in the lymph nodes, spleen and bone marrow (88). *H. canis* meronts are usually round to oval, about 30 μm in diameter, and include elongated micromerozoites with defined nuclei. A cross-section of the meront through the midshaft of the micromerozoites reveals a form with a central core mass surrounded by a circle of micromerozoite nuclei, which is often referred to as a 'wheel spoke' (76). This form is typical for HCI but is not found in HAI. Meronts of *H. canis* can sometimes be detected in tissues with little or no apparent host inflammatory response (89). This is possibly associated with the ability of the parasite to cause chronic subclinical infections and avoid an extreme immune response.

Cachexia and muscle atrophy are consistent gross findings on necropsy of dogs chronically infected with *H. americanum*. Roughening and thickening of bone surfaces may be apparent. Grossly, pyogranulomas may appear as multiple, 1–2 mm diameter, white-to-tan foci diffusely scattered throughout muscle and various other tissues. Microscopically, the cysts, meronts and pyogranulomas are found predominantly in skeletal and cardiac muscle but they may also be found sporadically in other tissues including adipose tissue, lymph node, intestinal smooth muscle, spleen, skin, kidney, salivary gland, liver, pancreas and lung. Vascular changes in various organs include fibrinoid degeneration of vessel walls, mineralization and proliferation of vascular intima and pyogranulomatous vasculitis. Renal lesions are frequently present and include focal pyogranulomatous inflammation with mild glomerulonephritis, lympho-plasmacytic interstitial nephritis, mesangioproliferative glomerulonephritis and, occasionally, amyloidosis. Amyloid deposits may also be found in spleen, lymph nodes, small intestines and liver. Occasional findings include pulmonary congestion, splenic coagulative necrosis, lymphadenopathy and congestion of the gastric mucosa.

Treatment and control

H. canis infection is treated with imidocarb dipropionate (5–6 mg/kg i/m every 14 days) until gamonts are no longer present in blood smears. Doxycyline (10 mg/kg p/o q24h for 21 days) is also used in combination with imidocarb dipropionate for treatment of HCI. The elimination of *H. canis* gamonts from the peripheral blood may require eight weeks, and a haematological evaluation every two weeks is indicated. Treatment is recommended for all infected dogs, including those with a mild disease, because parasitaemia may increase over time and develop into a severe infection. Generally, the survival

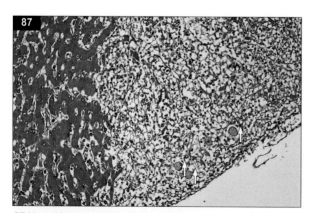

87 Hepatitis associated with *H. canis* meronts in a section of liver from a dog with a high parasitaemia. Arrows indicate the location of *H. canis* meronts.

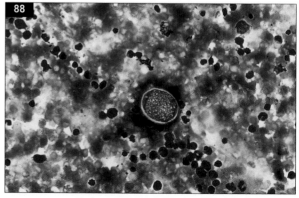

88 Developing *H. canis* meront in a cytological preparation from a bone marrow aspirate.

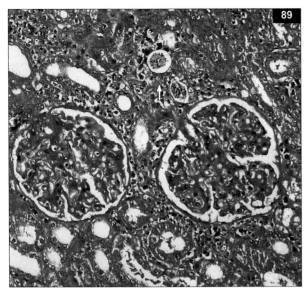

89 *H. canis* meront in kidney tissue. An arrow indicates the location of the meront. Meronts are often found with little or no surrounding inflammatory response.

Table 20 TCP treatment of *H. americanum* infection. These drugs are given in combination for 14 days and followed by long-term treatment with decoquinate.

Drug	Dose rate	Frequency of administration
Trimethoprim-sulphadiazine	15 mg/kg p/o	q12h
Clindamycin	10 mg/kg p/o	q8h
Pyrimethamine	0.25 mg/kg p/o	q24h

rate of dogs with a low *H. canis* parasitaemia is good. It is often dependent on the prognosis of any concurrent disease conditions. The prognosis for dogs with a high parasitaemia is less favourable. Seven of 15 dogs (47%) with a high parasitaemia included in the case-controlled study survived only two months after presentation despite specific treatment.

Both specific therapy using antiprotozoal drugs and palliative therapy using a non-steroidal anti-inflammatory drug (NSAID) have been used in the treatment of HAI. The best results occur when both are used together initially. An NSAID at standard doses can provide immediate relief from fever and pain during the first days of therapy before the effects of the antiprotozoal drug become evident.

Currently, it appears there is no drug capable of eliminating all stages of the organism. Remission of clinical signs can usually be obtained quickly by administering a combination of trimethoprim-sulphadiazine, clindamycin and pyrimethamine (TCP) for 14 days (*Table 20*). Although the clinical response is dramatic, it is often short-lived and most dogs relapse within 2–6 months following treatment.

The anticoccidial drug decoquinate helps prevent relapses when given daily to *H. americanum*-infected dogs after completion of TCP therapy. It likely arrests development of parasites released from mature meronts, thereby interrupting the repeated cycles of asexual reproduction. Decoquinate does not clear gamonts from the dog's circulation nor is it effective in reducing clinical signs associated with acute relapse. This drug must be

given every day to be effective. Although not approved for use in dogs, decoquinate has been proven to be safe in dogs at both high dosages and prolonged administration. The drug is available in the USA as a cornmeal-based premix for livestock at a concentration of 27.2 grams of decoquinate per pound of premix (Deccox, Alpharma Inc., Fort Lee, NJ). The powder is given at a rate of 0.5–1.0 teaspoonful per 10 kg body weight, mixed with moist dog food and fed twice daily. This amount corresponds to a decoquinate dosage of 10–20 mg/kg every 12 hours. It appears that the drug must be given long term (1–2 years and possibly longer) to prevent relapses.

In a study comparing treatment protocols, the two-year survival rate for dogs receiving only TCP was 12.5% compared to a two-year survival rate of greater than 84% when TCP was followed by long-term daily decoquinate therapy. Most dogs that received TCP alone had a very good initial response, followed by periodic relapses, resulting in chronic wasting and debilitation and ending in renal failure, euthanasia or death with a median survival time of approximately 12 months.

Control and prevention

Prevention of both HCI and HAI consists primarily of good tick control using an effective acaricide and close examination of dogs after hunting or outdoor activity. Dogs must be prevented from ingesting ticks. Until more is known about whether HCI or HAI can be transmitted through ingestion of infected tissues, dogs should also be prevented from eating raw meat or organs from wildlife and prevented from scavenging.

FELINE HEPATOZOONOSIS

Feline hepatozoonosis was first described in a domestic cat in 1908 in India, and has since been reported from several countries including France, Israel, South Africa, Brazil and Nigeria. The species of *Hepatozoon* that infect cats have not been identified and the vector is unknown. Gamonts of *Hepatozoon* are found in peripheral blood neutrophils (90) and histopathological studies have identified meronts in the myocardium and skeletal muscles of infected cats. In addition, in one retrospective study elevated CK levels have been found in the majority of cats with hepatozoonosis, indicating the importance of muscle as a target tissue for this infection. Feline hepatozoonosis is commonly associated with immunosuppressive viral disease caused by feline immunodeficiency virus or feline leukaemia virus.

ZOONOTIC POTENTIAL/PUBLIC HEALTH SIGNIFICANCE

There is only one report of human infection with a *Hepatozoon* species. Gamonts were found in the blood of a male patient from the Philippines on two different occasions but liver and bone marrow biopsies failed to reveal any parasites. Because canine hepatozoonosis occurs as a result of ingestion of a tick, transmission of *H. canis* or *H. americanum* to humans is unlikely except perhaps in small children inclined to put foreign objects into their mouths. Since other tick-borne diseases may be transmitted through the bite of a tick, all ticks should be promptly removed from any human or animal.

Disclaimer

The views expressed in this chapter are those of the authors and do not reflect the official policy or position of the Department of the Army, the Department of Defense, or the US Government.

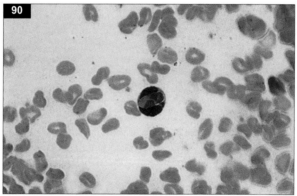

90 Gamont of an *Hepatozoon* species in a neutrophil of a naturally infected domestic cat.

8 Leishmaniosis

Gad Baneth, Michael Day, Xavier Roura and Susan Shaw

BACKGROUND, AETIOLOGY AND EPIDEMIOLOGY

Canine leishmaniosis is an important, potentially fatal disease that is also infectious to people. It is a part of a broad spectrum of diseases caused in humans and animals by several species of the intracellular protozoan genus *Leishmania* and is transmitted by sandflies. The disease syndromes caused by *Leishmania* species in people are cutaneous, mucocutaneous and visceral leishmaniosis, the last being the most severe form. Visceral leishmaniosis is further divided into zoonotic, in which dogs are reservoirs of the disease for people, and anthroponotic, in which man is the reservoir of infection for other humans and transmission by sandflies occurs without apparent involvement of an animal reservoir. *L. infantum* and *L. chagasi* cause zoonotic visceral leishmaniosis (ZVL), while anthroponotic infection is caused by *L. donovani*, mostly in India and East Africa. The two main groups of human patients at risk for ZVL are young children and HIV-positive patients. The domestic dog is considered the main reservoir for human ZVL infection and, more recently, dogs have also been incriminated as reservoirs for *Leishmania* species causing cutaneous and mucocutaneous leishmaniosis in South America. Infection among populations of wild canines such as foxes and jackals has been reported in the Mediterranean basin and South America and may also play a role in the epidemiology of ZVL in these regions.

ZVL transmission occurs in tropical, subtropical and temperate regions of the world including southern Europe, North and Central Africa, the Middle East, China and South and Central America (**91**). In the Mediterranean region and the Middle East, ZVL is caused by *L. infantum* and in South America by *L. chagasi*, which is thought to be synonymous with *L. infantum*. Canine leishmaniosis caused by *L. infantum* has also been recently reported from multiple kennels in the eastern USA, where the patterns of transmission are currently unknown. An additional *Leishmania* species, *L. tropica*, which is an agent of cutaneous leishmaniosis in the Old World that can visceralize in people, has been reported as a rare cause of canine visceral leishmaniosis in North Africa.

The prevalence rates of canine leishmaniosis in endemic areas vary depending on the environmental conditions required for transmission and the methods used for detecting infection. Seroprevalence rates in the Mediterranean basin range between 10% and 37% of the dogs in endemic foci. Surveys employing methods for the detection of leishmanial DNA in canine tissues, or combining serology and DNA detection, have revealed even higher infection rates approaching 70% in some foci. It is probable that all dogs living in endemic foci of leishmaniosis are exposed to infection and will develop either disease or subclinical infection, or resistance to infection.

91 The global distribution of canine leishmaniosis.

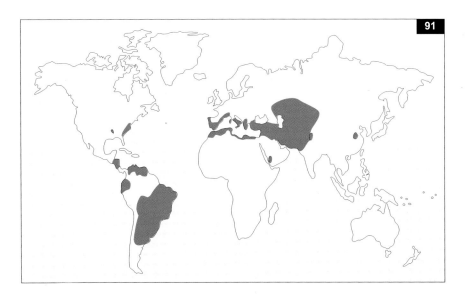

Leishmaniosis is now frequently diagnosed in countries where no sandfly transmission occurs in dogs; it is related to increased mobility of dogs and their owners. In Europe, many dogs travel to and from *Leishmania*-endemic areas and re-homing of stray animals from endemic areas by welfare groups is increasing the number of clinical cases seen in non-endemic areas. In addition, leishmaniosis is seen in non-travelled animals resident in non-endemic areas of both Europe and the USA. The mechanisms of transmission in these cases are currently unknown.

In contrast to dogs, natural infection and clinical disease in domestic cats caused by *Leishmania* species appear to be rare. Whether the low prevalence of infection/disease in endemic areas is due to under-reporting or to the fact that cats have a high degree of natural resistance is unknown. It has been shown that cats are relatively resistant to experimental infection with *L. chagasi* and *L. donovani*. However, cases of systemic clinical disease and asymptomatic infection due to *L. infantum* and other species are reported, and wild cats have been incriminated as reservoirs for leishmaniosis in endemic Mediterranean countries. Cutaneous lesions alone have been reported in association with *L. venezuelensis*, *L. mexicana*, *L. braziliensis* and unspecified *Leishmania* species in Europe and South America and in the southern USA.

Transmission and life cycle

Leishmania are diphasic parasites that complete their life cycle in two hosts: a vertebrate where the intracellular amastigote parasite forms are found, and a sandfly that harbours the flagellated extracellular promastigotes. Sandflies of the genus *Phlebotomus* are vectors in the Old World, whereas the vectors in the New World are sandflies of the genus *Lutzomyia*. The life cycle in both the reservoir host and vector is illustrated (**92**).

Although transmission of *L. infantum* occurs naturally by the bite of sandflies, vertical transmission *in utero* from dam to its offspring has been documented. Direct transmission without involvement of a haematophagous vector has been suspected in some cases of infection in areas where vectors of the disease are absent. Transmission of *L. infantum* by infected blood transfusion has been reported in dogs in North America and in human intravenous drug users sharing syringes in Spain.

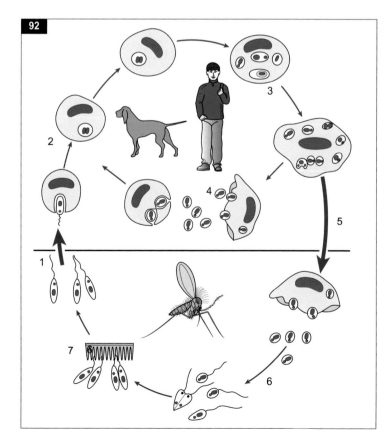

92 The life cycle of *Leishmania infantum* in the sandfly vector and its mammalian hosts (canines and man). (1) During a blood meal taken by the female sandfly, promastigotes are injected with saliva into the vertebrate host's skin. (2) and (3) Promastigotes are phagocytosed by macrophages in the skin and multiply by binary fission to amastigotes. (4) The macrophage ruptures and free amastigotes penetrate adjacent host cells and disseminate to the visceral organs. (5) Cells containing amastigotes are taken up by the sandfly during a blood meal. (6) Amastigotes are released from host cells, transform to promastigotes and multiply. (7) Promastigotes attach to the sandfly's gut wall where they continue to multiply and eventually reach the proboscis before infecting a naïve host.

PATHOGENESIS

Leishmaniosis is the classical example of a disease where the clinical signs and underlying pathology are intrinsically related to the interaction between the microbe, arthropod vector and host immune system. These interactions have been widely studied in both experimentally induced and spontaneously arising disease in a number of host species, and much of the current knowledge concerning the functional interactions between different T lymphocyte subpopulations was first established using murine models of this infection.

In susceptible animals, motile *Leishmania* promastigotes inoculated percutaneously by sandflies adhere rapidly to resident or recruited mononuclear phagocytes in the skin, using complement receptors. This is followed by rapid internalization of the parasite by phagocytosis and the transformation of promastigotes to non-motile amastigotes that are protected within the phagolysosome by low pH and the proteolytic activity of gp63 (**93**). Initially, a granulocytic infiltrate dominates the local cutaneous inflammatory response but this is followed by a macrophage and natural killer cell response. Later, lymphocytes appear and progression to a local granulomatous response occurs. Spread from the localized cutaneous lesion is a major event in the pathogenesis of visceral leishmaniosis. In susceptible animals, dissemination of infected macrophages to the local lymph node, spleen and bone marrow occurs within a few hours of inoculation. In resistant animals, parasites remain localized in the skin or at worst are restricted to the local lymph node. Susceptible animals once infected may remain asymptomatic for months to years and incubation periods as long as seven years have been reported.

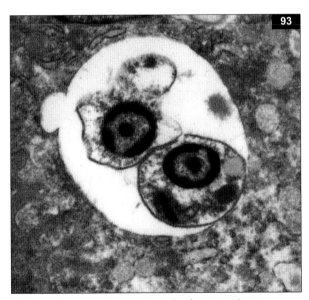

93 Transmission electron micrograph of a macrophage showing amastigote forms of *Leishmania* within a cytoplasmic compartment.

Immunopathogenesis

Leishmaniosis provides the single best example of polarization of the immune response to an infectious agent (see Chapter 3). Mice, humans and dogs generally develop chronic, progressive disease (a 'non-healing' phenotype) if the immune response is dominated by type 2 (Th2) immunity. In contrast, where immunity is dominated by a type 1 (Th1) response, dogs may become infected without developing clinical disease or develop disease that is mild and self-limiting. The mechanisms underlying this polarization are only just beginning to be understood. There is a clear genetic influence on the disease resistant, 'self-healing' phenotype. This has been shown in murine models and also likely holds true for the dog; for example, Ibizian Hounds have been shown to be relatively disease resistant. Resistance may relate to the early interactions between the organism and particular molecules expressed by antigen presenting cells of the immune system (e.g. pattern recognition molecules). An association between disease resistance and expression of a particular form of the gene encoding the molecule NRAMP1 (S1c11a1) has been investigated in mice, humans and dogs. The molecule encoded by this gene is an ion transporter involved in both macrophage activation and control of *Leishmania* replication within the cytoplasmic phagosome. The gene has been implicated in determining resistance or susceptibility to leishmaniosis in mice, and a recent study has suggested that mutations in this gene may control susceptibility in dogs. An association between susceptibility to leishmaniosis and specific allotypes of canine MHC class II (DLA) genes has also been recently defined.

More recent studies have suggested a role for populations of regulatory T lymphocytes (e.g. IL-10 producing Treg cells) in the pathogenesis of leishmaniosis. These Treg cells may inhibit the function of effector Th1 cells, thereby preventing complete elimination of the organisms and establishing persistent infection.

There is clear evidence in dogs of susceptible and resistant phenotypes with polarized immune responses. Susceptible animals mount significant antibody responses but have weak cell-mediated immunity. The reverse holds true for resistant dogs. These have reduced serological responses but strong intradermal responses to leishmanin and production of Th1-related cytokines (e.g. IFNγ) in response to antigen stimulation of lymphocyte cultures. Neutrophils and macrophages derived from *Leishmania*-infected dogs have reduced *in vitro* killing function. However, lymphocytes from resistant dogs co-cultured with infected macrophages exhibit strong intracellular killing of parasites. This killing is MHC class II restricted and is mediated by CD8+ and CD4+ T lymphocytes that produce the cytokine IFNγ. Immunohistochemical investigations of cutaneous lesions have shown reduced expression of MHC class II by epidermal Langerhans cells and keratinocytes and fewer infiltrating T lymphocytes within severe generalized nodular lesions, compared with milder alopecic dermatitis. There is debate in the canine literature as to whether there is an imbalance in the IgG subclass response to *Leishmania* in susceptible versus resistant dogs, and the variable results obtained in different studies may be a reflection of the quality of the immunological reagents used. A recent study has suggested that the serological response may not be clearly polarized, as elevation in all four IgG subclasses occurs during infection.

There is very little information on the immunological response to *Leishmania* infection in the cat. One cat with cutaneous leishmaniosis in southern Texas failed to respond to intradermal leishmanin injection, although other parameters of immune competence were reported as normal.

This immunological background helps explain the clinicopathological features of overt leishmaniosis as it presents in the dog. In animals that develop disseminated infection, lesions and clinical signs develop over a period of three months to several years after infection. Parasite-laden macrophages will accumulate in various sites of the body, particularly the lymphoid organs, producing generalized granulomatous lymphadenitis, splenomegaly and hepatomegaly. Extension of the disease process commonly leads to the development of granulomatous dermatitis, uveitis and infiltration of the bone marrow with infected macrophages. Case reports of leishmanial granulomatous lesions in a range of other sites (e.g. meninges, pericardium, intestine, muscle) have been published.

The dominance of type 2 (antibody-mediated) immunity in susceptible animals also has a role in the immunopathogenesis of disease. In such dogs there will be massive non-specific polyclonal activation of B-lymphocytes, with associated lymphoid follicular hyperplasia and serum hypergammaglobulinaemia. Occasionally, monoclonal gammopathy occurs, suggesting a more restricted activation of B cell clones. This excessive antibody production in turn produces cellular and tissue damage by evoking classical type II and type III hypersensitivity mechanisms, and the end effect is to mimic the clinical signs of multisystemic autoimmune disease. For example, immune-mediated haemolytic anaemia (Coombs test positive) and thrombocytopenia may occur in infected dogs as a consequence of aberrant antibody production. However, it is not clear whether this involves true autoantibody production triggered by the infection (perhaps by 'molecular mimicry') or the non-specific attachment of immune complexes to erythrocyte or platelet surfaces. Infected dogs may also be positive for serum antinuclear antibodies (ANA). Low ANA titres may simply reflect tissue damage in this disease but the occasional occurrence of high titres makes distinction from systemic lupus erythematosus important.

Leishmaniosis is an excellent example of an infectious disease that induces circulating immune complexes. At least some of the glomerulonephritis, uveitis and synovitis that characterize the systemic infection likely relates to vascular deposition of these complexes. For example, granular and diffuse IgG deposition has been recorded within the granulomatous uveal tract lesions of infected dogs, together with evidence of vasculitis and thrombosis. Similar immunohistochemical studies have demonstrated immunoglobulin deposition within the glomerular lesions of infected dogs. Again, the antigenic content of these complexes has not been investigated in the canine disease.

The complex immunopathological mechanisms that underlie the clinical features of *Leishmania* infection may be further complicated in cases of co-infection with other arthropod-borne agents such as *Babesia* or *Ehrlichia* species. For details of pathogenic mechanisms in these diseases see Chapters 6 and 11, respectively.

Table 21 Frequency of clinical signs occurring in a large canine leishmaniosis case series (>100 animals) from Italy and Greece. (After Ciaramella *et al.*, 1997; Koutinas *et al.*, 1999)

Clinical signs	Relative frequency of occurrence (%)
Lymphadenopathy	65.2–88.7
Cutaneous involvement	56.0–81.0
Pale mucous membranes	58.0
Splenomegaly	9.5–53.3
Weight loss	25.3–32.0
Abnormal claws	24.0–30.5
Ocular involvement	16.0–24.1
Anorexia	16.5–18.0
Epistaxis	3.8–10.0
Lameness	3.3
Diarrhoea	3.0–3.8

Table 22 Frequency of cutaneous findings occurring in canine leishmaniosis cases (*n* = 22) from Greece. (After Koutinas *et al.*, 1993)

Dermatological signs	Relative frequency of occurrence (%)
Exfoliative dermatitis	90.9
Ulceration	63.6
Generalized hypotrichosis, especially face and pinnae	59.1
Abnormal claws	54.5
Focal alopecia (pinnae and face)	50.0
Mild to moderate pruritus	18.2
Paronychia	13.6

CLINICOPATHOLOGICAL FINDINGS

Dogs

Clinical canine leishmaniosis has a chronic waxing and waning course. Commonly, there is a history of non-specific illness combined with lymphadenomegaly, cutaneous signs, weight loss, splenomegaly and pale mucous membranes (*Table 21*). Cutaneous signs are of major importance in this disease and include exfoliative dermatitis, which produces a characteristic silvery scale that is prominent on the face, periocular region and pinnae; periocular alopecia; and abnormal growth of claws (*Table 22*) (**94–97**). Ulcerative and nodular dermatitis may occur secondary to vasculitis and granulomatous inflammation (**94–97**).

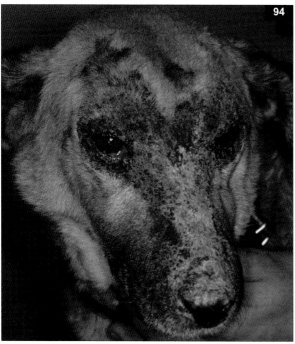

94 Crossbred dog showing facial alopecia, crusting and ulceration. In addition, there is depigmentation and ulceration of the nasal planum.

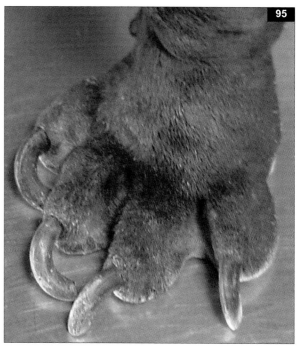

95 Pododermatitis with scaling, paronychia and onychogryphosis in a dog with leishmaniosis.

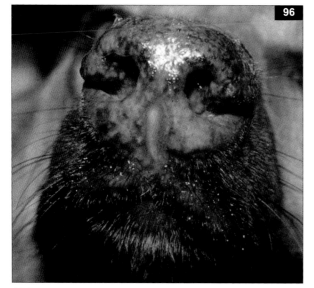

96 Depigmentation, erosion, ulceration and loss of cobblestone pattern of the planum nasale in a dog with leishmaniosis.

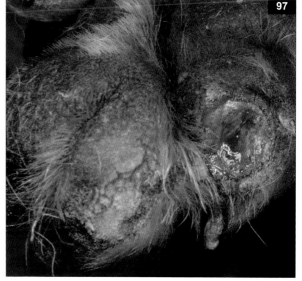

97 Central foot pad ulceration secondary to granulomatous dermatitis and/or vasculitis in a dog with leishmaniosis.

Ocular and periocular signs are frequently seen in canine leishmaniosis (*Table 23*) (**98, 99**). Less commonly, lameness due to arthropathies, diarrhoea and epistaxis are reported (*Table 21*, p. 92) (**100**). Although multisystemic disease is characteristic of leishmaniosis, affected dogs may present with clinical signs referable to one body system only. There are reports of infections associated with colitis, myositis, osteomyelitis and arthrosynovitis, as well as isolated ocular disease.

Clinical laboratory findings are dominated by high globulin levels due to massive gammaglobulin production, and a monoclonal or biclonal gammopathy may be seen (*Table 24*) (**101**). Hypoalbuminaemia, predominantly due to protein-losing glomeru-lonephropathy, is also a common finding. Anaemia is frequently identified and is often Coombs positive. Affected dogs are commonly ANA positive. Thrombocytopenia and haemostatic abnormalities have been reported with varying frequency in cases of canine leishmaniosis. However, although prolonged bleeding times are consistently found in infected dogs, reports disagree as to the frequency and cause of thrombocytopenia. Both antibody-mediated destruction and disseminated intravascular coagulation have been suggested. In addition, co-infection with *Ehrlichia* and *Anaplasma* species (see Chapter 11) should be eliminated in cases with bleeding tendencies. Concurrent *Ehrlichia canis* seropositivity was found in 14% of 150 Italian cases of leishmaniosis. Reported co-infection with sarcoptic or demodectic mange and hepatozoonosis may be coincidental.

Cats

The pathogenesis of the disease in cats has not been investigated. The clinical presentation is similar to that seen in dogs, although the small number of cases makes the association of infection and clinical signs difficult to interpret. Cutaneous lesions include diffuse areas of alopecia and granulomatous dermatitis of the head, scaling and pinnal dermatitis, ulceration and nodules. Systemic involvement with *L. infantum* has been reported in association with jaundice, vomiting, hepatomegaly, splenomegaly, lymphadenomegaly, membranous glomerulonephritis and granulomatous gastroenteritis. In the small number of cases investigated, association with the immunosuppressive viruses (FIV or FeLV) has not been confirmed.

DIAGNOSIS

Confirming a diagnosis of leishmaniosis in an individual case may be difficult, particularly if the clinical signs are not specific. In addition, longitudinal studies of *Leishmania* infection show that relative predictive values for diagnostic tests vary depending on the stage of infection. Consequently, a diagnostic approach that involves multiple testing is recommended and no single diagnostic technique identifies all infected animals.

Table 23 Frequency of ocular and periocular findings occurring in canine leishmaniosis cases (n = 105) from Spain. (After Pena *et al.*, 2000)

Ophthalmological signs	Relative frequency of occurrence (%)
Anterior uveitis	42.8
Conjunctivitis	31.4
Keratoconjunctivitis	31.4
Blepharitis	29.5
Periocular alopecia	26.7
Posterior uveitis	3.8
Keratoconjunctivitis sicca	2.8
Orbital cellulitis	1.9

Table 24 Frequency of clinical laboratory findings occurring in a large canine leishmaniosis case series (n = 150) from Italy. (After Ciaramella *et al.*, 1997)

Clinical laboratory signs	Relative frequency of occurrence (%)
Hyperglobulinaemia	70.6
Hypoalbuminaemia	68.0
Anaemia	58.0
Positive ANA	52.8
Neutrophila	24.0
Thrombocytopenia	29.3
Positive Coombs test	20.8
Azotaemia	16.0
Elevated liver enzymes	16.0

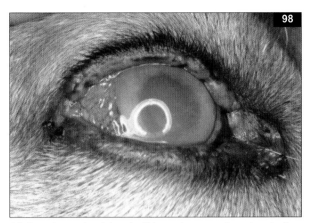

98 Granulomas involving the lid margins, granulomatous bulbar conjunctivitis and corneal opacity in a dog with leishmaniosis.

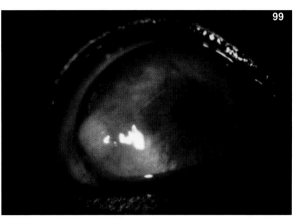

99 Corneal granulomatous infiltrate with uveitis in a dog with leishmaniosis.

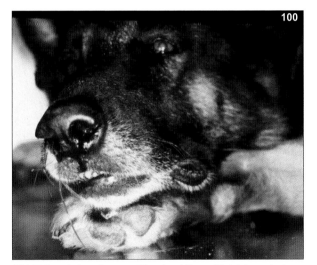

100 Epistaxis in a German Shepherd Dog with leishmaniosis.

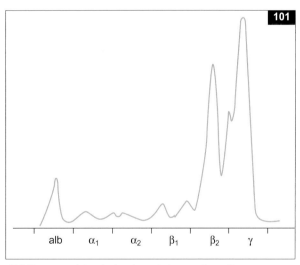

101 Serum protein electrophoresis from a dog with leishmaniosis, showing a biclonal gammopathy.

Microscopic identification of organisms or their DNA

Intracellular or extracellular *Leishmania* amastigotes can be identified in Giemsa- or Leishmans-stained tissue aspirates and impression or biopsy samples from lymph node, conjunctiva, bone marrow (**102**), spleen and lesional skin (**103, 104**). Amastigotes are small round or oval bodies 1.5–3.0 × 2.5–3.5 μm in size and without a free flagellum. The organism has a relatively large nucleus and a kinetoplast. However, the sensitivity of microscopic examination is relatively poor (60%) as more than 50% of lymph node and bone marrow samples have low parasite density. PCR targeting kinetoplast DNA, and immunohistochemical techniques for increasing sensitivity and specificity of *Leishmania* detection, have been developed for use in fresh and frozen bone marrow, lymph node and skin biopsy specimens (**105**). On such samples the sensitivity of PCR approaches 95–100%. However, the sensitivity of PCR on peripheral blood samples is highest shortly after infection (88%) and then decreases with chronicity and tissue sequestration of the organism to 50–70%.

Serology

Most dogs with visceral leishmaniosis develop a specific humoral immune response and serodiagnostic testing is widely used. However, specificity is decreased in Central and South America due to cross-reactivity with trypanosomes. The sensitivity of serology is lowest (41%) early in *Leishmania* infection (first few months) but high with progressive infection (93–100%). Sensitivity may also be limited in cases of localized cutaneous leishmanial infection. A wide variety of serological assays are available, utilizing indirect immunofluorescence (IFA), direct agglutination, conventional ELISA, dot-ELISA, competitive ELISA and western blotting methodology. Although there is some variation in specificity, sensitivity and predictive values, most are acceptable. At present most tests employ crude *Leishmania* antigen, although a recombinant *Leishmania* K39 ELISA has been recently validated. Several rapid immunochromatographic test kits have also been produced for canine leishmaniosis but although most are relatively specific, sensitivity varies from 35–76%.

Culture and species characterization

Culture can be used for diagnosis of canine *Leishmania* infection but it requires access to a laboratory with technical expertise and appropriate containment facilities. In addition, multiple samples are required from several sites to achieve appropriate sensitivity. It is, however, the basis for species characterization using traditional isoenzyme analysis and molecular techniques such as random amplification of polymorphic DNA (RAPD). However, as primer sequences for differentiation of New and Old World species are now available, PCR and sequencing are commonly used.

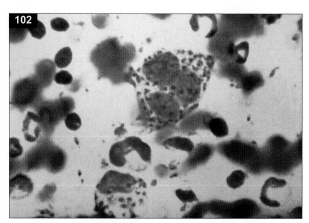

102 Bone marrow aspirate from dog with leishmaniosis, showing intracellular *Leishmania* amastigotes.

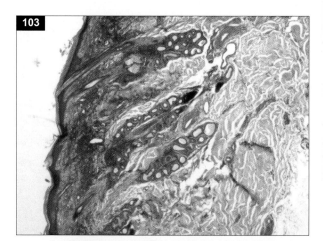

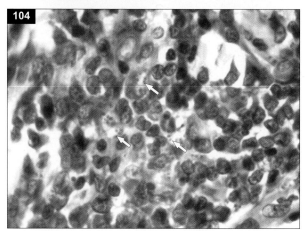

103, 104 Skin biopsy from a dog with leishmaniosis. There are numerous infiltrating macrophages in the superficial dermis, within which *Leishmania* amastigotes (**104**, arrows) can be clearly seen.

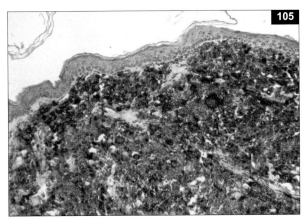

105 Immunohistochemical labelling of skin biopsy from dog with leishmaniosis to demonstrate the presence of amastigotes. (Photo courtesy Department of Pathology, Veterinary Faculty, Universitat Autònoma de Barcelona)

TREATMENT AND CONTROL

Chemotherapeutic treatment of canine leishmaniosis

Several drugs are currently used for the treatment of canine leishmaniosis (*Table 25*). Therapy with these drugs often achieves clinical improvement in dogs but rarely is it associated with elimination of parasite carriage or the prevention of clinical disease relapse. Special consideration must be taken prior to therapy if the patient has impaired renal or hepatic function.

Antimonials have been used for the therapy of leishmaniosis since the early 20th century, when tartar emetic (antimony potassium tartrate) was adapted for the treatment of human leishmaniosis in South America after proving effective against African trypanosomiasis. Pentavalent antimonials are still widely used against the different forms of leishmaniosis in both human and

Table 25 Drugs used for therapy of leshmaniosis.

Drug	Common trade name	Class	Mode of action	Therapeutic protocol	Adverse effects
Meglumine antimonate	Glucantime	Pentavalent antimonial	Inhibition of enzymes active in glycolysis and fatty acid oxidation	100 mg/kg s/c for 3–4 weeks	Nephrotoxicity, pain and muscle fibrosis at the site of injection
Allopurinol	Zyloric	Pyrazolpyrimidine	Incorporation into RNA and inhibition of protein synthesis	(**1**) 20 mg/kg p/o q24h indefinitely (**2**) 20 mg/kg p/o q24h combined with meglumine antimonate (100 mg/kg s/c q24h for 20 days), continued with allopurinol alone (20 mg/kg q24h indefinitely)	Xanthine urolith formation
Amphotericin B	Fungizone	Polyene macrolide	Alteration of membrane permability by binding to ergosterol	(**1**) For free amphotericin B: 0.5–0.8 mg/kg i/v or s/c 2–3 times a week until an accumulated dose of 15 mg/kg is reached (**2**) For administration in lipid emulsion: 1.0–2.5 mg/kg i/v mixed in lipid emulsion twice a week until an accumulated dose of 10 mg/kg is reached	Nephrotoxicity
	AmBisome (liposomalized)			(**3**) For liposomalized amphotericin B: 3 mg/kg/day i/v until a total dose of 15 mg/kg is reached	

veterinary medicine. The antimonials selectively inhibit leishmanial enzymes that are required for glycolytic and fatty acid oxidation. Meglumine antimonate is the principal antimonial used as monotherapy or in combination with other drugs for the treatment of dogs. The reports of *L. infantum* strains that are resistant to pentavalent antimonials are of major veterinary and public health concern.

Allopurinol is an orally administered purine analogue that is metabolized by *Leishmania* parasites and incorporated in RNA, causing an interruption in protein synthesis. The relative non-toxicity, clinical efficacy, low cost and convenience of oral administration have made allopurinol a popular choice for the treatment of canine leishmaniosis. It is recommended as daily treatment for an indefinite period of time and is commonly administered in combination or following initial therapy with meglumine antimonate. The combination of allopurinol and meglumine antimonate allows a decrease in the duration of meglumine therapy, making it better tolerated and less costly. In addition, long-term therapy with allopurinol decreases the rate of relapse after meglumine antimonate treatment.

Amphotericin B is a polyene macrolide that is mostly used as an anti-fungal drug but which also has activity against some protozoal species. It acts by binding to ergosterol and altering cell membrane permeability. Amphotericin B has a toxic effect on the canine kidney, which is mediated by renal vasoconstriction and subsequent reduction of the glomerular filtration rate, and possibly also by direct action on renal epithelial cells. It can be administered to dogs with leishmaniosis in its highly nephrotoxic-free form, in a lipid emulsion, or in a liposomal formulation that reduces its toxic effects and enhances penetration of the drug into macrophages and its accumulation in visceral organs.

Another drug that has been evaluated for canine leishmaniosis is pentamidine, an aromatic diamidine used also for pneumocystosis, babesiosis and trypanosomiasis. It is injected intramuscularly in dogs and can cause severe irritation at the site of injection, hypotension, tachycardia and vomiting. Other drugs that have been used or are being investigated for the treatment of canine leishmaniosis include aminosidine, alkylphosphocholine derivatives, metronidazole and ketoconazole.

The diagnosis and treatment of concurrent diseases such as ehrlichiosis and babesiosis may be required, as these infections are common in areas of *L. infantum* endemnicity.

The prognosis for canine leishmaniosis depends on the severity of organ injury at the time of diagnosis. In dogs that are not in renal failure, treatment frequently achieves dramatic improvement in both cutaneous and systemic signs of the disease and limits progression of the disease. However, as mentioned previously, there are no treatment protocols published that result in parasitological cure. Consequently, if treatment is discontinued, the chance of disease recrudescence is high even if the clinical response was excellent.

Vaccination

The development of an effective vaccine for canine leishmaniosis remains a major challenge for the control of this zoonotic infection in endemic areas and is an active area of research. The enormous knowledge of the immune response to this infection provides an excellent platform for such vaccine development, and there is a large literature on the application of various vaccine candidates in murine models. Clearly, an effective vaccine requires induction of a strong protective type 1 (Th1) immune response in susceptible animals. For this to be achieved there must be selection of the most appropriate antigenic components of the organism, and the delivery of these to the canine population in conjunction with an adjuvant system that optimally stimulates type 1 immunity. Numerous studies have demonstrated seropositivity to a wide range of *Leishmania* antigens in infected dogs and shown how the range of antigens recognized changes throughout the course of infection.

There have been relatively few studies of vaccination against leishmaniosis performed in dogs. Dogs administered entire *Leishmania* promastigotes with BCG developed strong lymphocyte proliferative responses but low antibody titre, in comparison with dogs administered the same antigen in saponin, and a protective effect upon challenge was shown. A field study using *L. donovani* fucose mannose ligand (FML) in Quil A saponin demonstrated induction of protective cell-mediated immunity by vaccination. Not all studies have had a successful outcome. Dogs vaccinated with a 67–94 kDa antigen derived from *L. infantum* promastigotes had a higher rate of infection and clinical disease than controls, suggesting that this vaccine may have induced non-protective Th2 immunity.

Such approaches are relatively crude in terms of current approaches to vaccination, and it would seem likely that development of a molecular vaccine ('naked DNA' or plasmid vaccine) using molecular adjuvants (e.g. CpG motifs or cytokine genes) would be a logical progression of these studies.

Other control methods

Efforts to control the spread of the disease in the canine population have, in general, not been successful. Medical treatment is targeted only at individual symptomatic dogs and is not even effective in eliminating the infection from these animals. The killing of seropositive sick dogs as exercised in South America is both unacceptable to the owners and not effective, because asymptomatic dogs and wild animal species serve as a source of parasite transmission. Chemical control by spraying insecticides against sandfly vectors is of limited effectiveness and may be harmful to the environment. A collar impregnated with the pyrethroid deltamethrin is manufactured for the protection of dogs from sandfly bites and appears to decrease the rate of infection among dogs and humans in endemic regions. The collar is effective against *Phlebotomus* and *Lutzomyia* species and is indicated for protection of dogs residing in or travelling to disease foci. Spot-on or spray products containing pyrethroids and/or other chemicals that repel sandflies are available for direct application onto dogs.

ZOONOTIC POTENTIAL/PUBLIC HEALTH SIGNIFICANCE

Visceral leishmaniosis is a potentially fatal disease, with 500,000 new human cases annually and a population at risk of 200 million people, as estimated by the World Health Organization (WHO) in a report from 1999. Anthroponotic visceral leishmaniosis caused by *L. donovani*, mainly in India and Sudan, is responsible for a large proportion of the fatalities in people. However, zoonotic visceral leshmaniosis, with the dog as a major reservoir for the parasite, is a main concern in other parts of the world including northeastern Brazil and southern Europe. The major risk group for human disease caused by *L. infantum* has traditionally been infants and children. Malnutrition has long been recognized as a risk factor for infantile leishmaniosis and this may explain why the disease is more prevalent among children in poor countries, compared with children in more affluent areas, which have a similar high prevalence rate in the dog population.

With the appearance of the AIDS epidemic, HIV-positive patients are now the predominant group of patients in southern Europe. The co-infection of HIV and leishmaniosis reported from more than 33 countries where these infections geographically overlap has been described as a 'deadly gridlock' that does not respond well to therapy and is ultimately fatal. HIV-positive patients are sensitive to new infection or a reactivation of a present dormant infection. The presence of large numbers of parasites in their tissues and blood makes them highly infectious to sandflies.

Keeping and treating infected dogs presents a dilemma to owners, veterinarians and public health officials in areas where suitable vectors are found, because of the risk of transmission to other people and pets in the community. Before deciding on therapy, owners must receive a thorough and realistic explanation about the disease, its zoonotic potential and the prognosis for their dog and what should be expected from treatment.

9 **Borreliosis**
K Emil Hovius

AETIOLOGY AND EPIDEMIOLOGY

Aetiology

Spirochaetes comprising the genus *Borrelia* are vector-transmitted bacteria of the order Spirochaetales. The specialized, elongated structure of these bacteria enables an undulating motility in environments of high viscosity such as the intercellular matrix of skin (**106**). The eleven described species in the *Borrelia burgdorferi* complex are transmitted by hard ticks, primarily *Ixodes* species (*Table 26*). Only three *Borrelia* species, *B. burgdorferi sensu stricto*, *B. garinii* and *B. afzelii*, are clinically important in humans and dogs. The other frequently encountered species, *Borrelia valaisiana*, *B. lusitanea* and *B. japonica*, are probably not of great clinical importance. Avian and bovine borreliosis, caused by *B. anserina* and *B. theileri*, respectively, are transmitted by *Argas* and *Boophilus* ticks. *Borrelia* species are also associated with relapsing fever in humans: *B. recurrentis* is louse borne while *B. hermsii* is transmitted by soft ticks of the genus *Ornithodorus*.

Epidemiology of the *Borrelia burgdorferi* complex

Many wild mammals and birds are known reservoirs for *Borrelia burgdorferi* species. The range of these is discussed fully in Chapter 2 and summarized in **107**.

European *Ixodes* species ticks may harbour co-infections of up to four different *Borrelia* species. Generally, *B. afzelii* appears to be most prevalent, although *B. valaisiana* may occur locally in the UK and Ireland and *B. garinii* occurs in some localized areas in Europe and Asia. In addition, even where one genotype predominates, infections with different strains of differing pathogenicity occur. Where strain variation exists, one tick bite may result in heterogeneous infection. There is pronounced strain variability of *B. garinii* isolated from ticks, which may be induced by the dispersing capabilities of the reservoir birds. Nymphal ticks play a central role in *B. burgdorferi* transmission and may even have a reservoir function. Their greatest abundance is in spring.

Dogs are capable of maintaining *Borrelia* infection; however, their role in the sylvatic cycle is limited. The

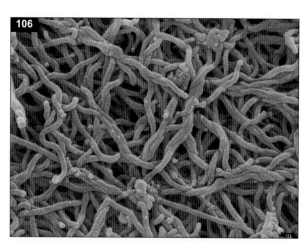

106 Scanning electron microscope image of *Borrelia burgdorferi* organisms. The image shows typical clustering of spirochaetes in Barbour–Stoenner–Kelly (BSK) liquid culture medium. The unique bipolar orientated flagellum of the spirochaetes is encapsulated by the outer surface envelope, enabling the slender protoplasmic cylinder to coil. (Electronmicrograph courtesy of Dr R Straubinger and Dr S Al-Robaiy, Institute for Immunology, and Prof J Seeger and Dr J Kacza, Institute for Histology and Embryology, College of Veterinary Medicine, University of Leipzig)

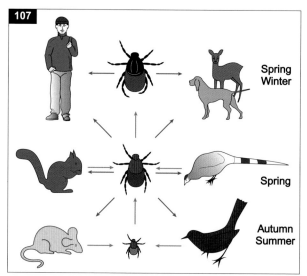

107 The cycle of *Borrelia* spirochaetes through the tick vector and vertebrate hosts. The European situation with mammalian and avian species is depicted, emphasizing the central role of the nymph. During the two-year tick life cycle the successive stages acquire or transmit spirochaetes by feeding on successively larger hosts. Birds are reservoirs for *B. garinii* and *B. valaisiana*. Small mammals are the reservoir animals for *B. burgdorferi sensu stricto* and *B. valaisiana*.

Table 26 Distribution, vectors and clinical relevance of the major *Borrelia* species. *B. burgdorferi sensu stricto* is the main species present in the USA. Its distribution is mainly in the northeastern and mid-western states, where it is transmitted by *Ixodes scapularis*, and in the south-west where it is transmitted by *I. pacificus*. In Europe, *B. burgdorferi sensu stricto* is transmitted by *I. ricinus*. *B. burgdorferi sensu stricto* does not survive in *I. persulcatus* and therefore is not found in Asia. The occurrence of *B. burgdorferi sensu stricto* in the Old World and in the New World has been explained by post-Columbus migrations. *B. garinii* is probably the most widespread species, with a range extending from western Europe to Japan. It is transported by migratory thrushes through European and Asian countries, and has great strain diversity. It is also carried from the northern to the southern hemisphere by sea birds carrying *I. uriae*. However, *B. garinii* is not detected in humans or in domestic animal species from the southern hemisphere. More species are being identified (e.g. the Florida canine spirochaete, an unknown *Borrelia* causing disease in dogs in Florida).

Lyme *Borrelia* species	Main vector	Main reservoirs	Distribution	Human disease	Canine infection	Canine disease
B. burgdorferi sensu stricto	*I. ricinus, I. scapularis, I. pacificus*	Rodents/birds	N. America, western Europe	N. America, Europe	N. America, Europe	N. America Europe
B. bisettii	*I. pacificus, I. scapularis*	Rodents	USA	No	No	No
B. andersonii	*I. dentatus*	Lizards	USA	No	No	No
B. afzelii	*I. ricinus, I. persulcatus, I. hexagonus*	Mainly rodents	Euroasia	Europe	Europe	Europe
B. garinii	*I. ricinus, I. persulcatus, I. uriae*	Mainly birds	Euroasia	Europe	Europe, Japan	Europe, Japan
B. valaisiana	*I. ricinus, I. columnae*	Mainly birds	Euroasia	Uncertain	Europe	Uncertain
B. lusitaniae	*I. ricinus, I. persulcatus*	Not well known	South-central Europe	No	No	No
B. japonica	*I. ovatus*	Rodents	Japan	No	Japan	Japan
B. sinica	*I. ovatus*	Rodents	South China	Unknown	Unknown	Unknown
B. tanukii	*I. tanuki*	Birds	Japan	No	No	No
B. turdae	*I. turdus*	Birds	Japan	No	No	No

reservoir competency of cats is currently unknown. Serological surveys of dogs for *B. burgdorferi* complex have been used as an indicator for infection rates in the local tick and wild animal populations and, thus, as an indication of risk for human infection. In Europe, 20–40% of questing (un-fed) ticks collected from the coat of dogs, or from vegetation in woods where dogs will walk, contain *Borrelia* DNA. Consequently, seropositivity rates for European dogs from wooded areas approximate 100%, and serological conversion in pups and rising titres in young dogs may occur during the tick seasons. In Westchester county, New York, 80% of questing ticks may contain borreliae and surveys of dogs in the northeastern USA reveal high levels (30–90%) of seropositivity.

In North America, *B. burgdorferi sensu stricto* is the only pathogenic species found in dogs. In Japan, dogs are probably infected with *B. japonica* and *B. garinii*. In Europe, dogs are mainly infected with *B. burgdorferi sensu stricto* and *B. garinii*, even in areas where ticks

carry multiple *Borrelia* species. This implies differences in infectivity and invasiveness of species and strains with respect to the canine host, and this phenomenon requires further investigation. The differential tissue tropism that the three species exert in the human host – *B. afzelii* to skin, *B. garinii* to the CNS and *B. burgdorferi sensu stricto* to synovial tissues – implies that differences in tissue affinity in the canine host might also be expected.

Longitudinal studies have shown that all dogs in an endemic area become infected. However, most dogs remain asymptomatic, with moderate serum antibody titres, while only a small percentage (approximately 5%) develop disease concurrent with a steep rise in titre. In addition, persistence of moderate serum antibody titres is not associated with clinical disease. However, dogs with heterogeneous infections or co-infections with other tick-transmitted pathogens (*Ehrlichia*, *Anaplasma*, *Bartonella*, *Babesia* and/or *Rickettsia* species) may be more likely to develop clinical borreliosis than dogs infected with a single *Borrelia* strain.

Information on feline *Borrelia* infection is sparse. In a serological survey of cats in the northeastern USA, 20% had antibodies against *B. burgdorferi*. In a UK study, 4.2% of cats were positive compared to more than 20% of dogs. None of these seropositive cats had clinical disease attributable to infection with the spirochaete. At present, the species naturally infecting cats are unknown.

PATHOGENESIS

Different mechanisms are exploited by borreliae to avoid clearance by the immune system, resulting in a persistent infection and possibly chronic disease (**108**, *Table 27*). The *Borrelia* genome is unusual compared to that of other bacteria, as it has a linear chromosome and an extraordinary number (21) of circular and linear

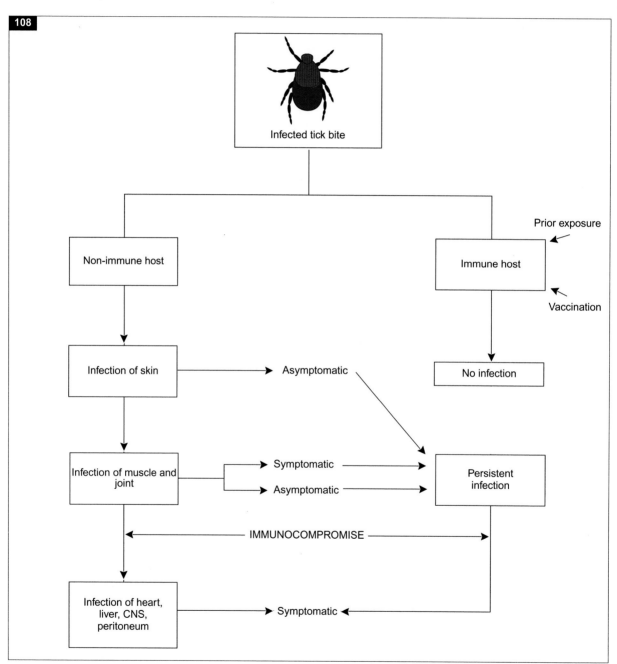

108 Possible outcome of *Borrelia* infection. If an infected tick bites an immune host, infection will not establish and the animal will remain asymptomatic. Transmission of borreliae to a non-immune host will allow the establishment of progressive infection in skin and then muscle and joints. This infection may be either symptomatic or asymptomatic and is likely to be persistent. Immunocompromise is likely to result in further spread of the infection, with the development of progressive clinical signs.

plasmids. The chromosome has been completely sequenced and is thought to contain only around 800 genes encoding molecules with metabolic functions. Many genes encoding molecules with metabolic functions normally present in bacterial genomes are missing, suggesting that borreliae are highly dependent on the host for metabolism. *Borrelia* species are not dependent on iron, which is possibly an adaptation to localization within connective tissue with limited access to the bloodstream. A large portion of the genome encodes molecules involved in motility, indicating the importance of migration in pathogenesis.

The plasmids encode around 100 proteins, of which the majority are lipoproteins located on the outer surface envelope in direct contact with the host. Six outer surface proteins, OspA to OspF, have been characterized, and these are highly immunogenic and antigenically variable. OspA (31–34 kDa) has been typed serologically, and seven serotypes are defined and assigned to three groups corresponding to the three pathogenic *B. burgdorferi* species. OspB (34–36 kDa) is highly conserved among the three pathogenic species and in isolates from different geographical regions. Four phenotypes of the many Osp C (20–24 kDa) genotypes are considered virulence factors, as their presence correlates with the capacity for visceral spread of infection. The change in expression from OspA to OspC on the outer envelope (the 'OspA/OspC switch') is mandatory for infection of the vertebrate host. This occurs within the first 48 hours of tick attachment. The expression of OspA is down-regulated by first contact with blood, and OspC is expressed as spirochaetes migrate from the tick midgut to the tick salivary gland. Consequently, OspC antibodies are detected in early infection of man and experimental animals, whereas OspA antibodies only occur in later stages of disease. Antibodies to OspA, OspB and OspC do not exert bactericidal activity within the infected host but prevent reinfection by killing borreliae in the presence of host blood complement in the tick gut.

The large potential for antigenic variation and immune evasion within the *Borrelia* species is due to recombination of numerous redundant gene copies found in the variable membrane protein-like system (vlsE) encoding for the vlsE surface lipoprotein. The vlsE antigen, although hypervariable, has fixed invariate regions that are conserved within all *Borrelia* species, making it a useful target for serodiagnosis.

The key component of the *Borrelia* flagellum, the 41 kDa flagellin protein, is highly immunogenic. Antibody directed to flagellin cross-reacts with other flagellated bacteria such as *Treponema* and *Leptospira* species. However, the variable central domain of the flagellin molecule is conserved within the genus *Borrelia*, rendering it a useful antigenic target for detecting specific antibodies. Antibodies directed at certain domains of the flagellin molecule may cross-react with neuroaxonal proteins, causing neuroborreliosis.

Immunocompetent host species studied, including rats, mice, hamsters, dogs and humans, tend to develop persistent infection without clinical manifestations. For example, experimental infection of hamsters results in persistent cardiac and urinary tract infection without clinical signs or histological changes. Immunosuppression is required for persistently infected animals to develop clinical disease. Susceptibility of laboratory mice to borreliosis is strain-dependent and related to the nature of the CD4+ T cell response to the organism (see Chapter 3).

In experimental canine infection, a single exposure to infected ticks results in active disease in very young animals only. In one study, beagle puppies (6–12 weeks of age) were infected by ticks harbouring *B. burgdorferi sensu stricto*. Two to five months after tick exposure the

Table 27 Possible disease phases of borreliosis in the dog. The disease phase (outcome) is determined by spirochaete numbers. The status of the immune system, reflected by the whole cell ELISA antibody titre, was inferred from experimental and natural infections. The clinical outcome of a *Borrelia* infection is dependent on an intricate balance between the immune system and the infecting strain.

Disease state (outcome)	Status of immune system	Titre whole cell ELISA	Spirochaetes in tissues
Permanent asymptomatic	Clears the spirochaetes or in balance with the spirochaetes	Very low to moderate titre	None or very low numbers
Acute and subacute disease	Immune suppression	Rise of titre to high values	Very high numbers
Chronic (intermittent) disease	Differentiates towards Th1 instead of Th2-response	Permanent high (fluctuating) levels	Fluctuating but high numbers
Convalescent	Clears the spirochaetes	Reverses to very low titres	None

pups developed mild clinical disease characterized by transient fever, behavioural changes and lameness. Approximately 50% of the animals had recurrent episodes of disease. After four months, clinical signs abated but infection and high serum antibody titres persisted. By contrast, adult dogs do not develop clinical disease after a single exposure to *Borrelia*-infected ticks. However, after 70 days of continuous or intermittent exposure to infected ticks, adult dogs develop mild clinical signs. Affected joint capsules contain spirochaetes and there is IL-8 production within the synovial membrane and chemotactic attraction of neutrophils into the joint. After several months of persistent infection, a mild subclinical polysynovitis occurs, with lymphoplasmacytic infiltration of the synovial membrane.

Quantitative PCR has been used to monitor infectious load in the tissues of dogs experimentally infected with *B.*

burgdorferi sensu stricto (*Table 28*). Skin and joint capsule taken from symptomatic dogs four months after infection contain many more spirochaetes than those from infected asymptomatic dogs. Symptomatic dogs also have a higher serum antibody titre. In this model, disease is self-limiting and the convalescent stage is characterized by a delicate balance achieved between the spirochaete and the host immune system. When this balance is disturbed, spirochaete numbers increase in the skin again, antibody titres rise and clinical signs may recur. If the symptomatic dogs are treated with appropriate antibiotics, spirochaete numbers decrease more rapidly than when convalescent. However, in some cases, several months post-antibiotic therapy (especially when glucocorticoids are used concurrently), *Borrelia* DNA can again be detected and antibody titres rise, indicating survival of the agent despite therapy.

Table 28 Presence of *Borrelia burgdorferi* in the tissues of symptomatic dogs. *B. burgdorferi sensu stricto* as a single agent in experimental infection (first 3 columns) may have a different tissue tropism (fibrous tissues) compared with *B. garinii* (liver) given as a coinfection with *B. burgdorferi sensu stricto* to European dogs (last column). Skin, lymph node, fascia, muscle and joint capsule consistently become infected by active migration along connective tissue planes. It is possible that this migratory route extends through the thoracic and abdominal wall and reaches the peritoneum and pericardial tissues, which in experimental infections frequently contain *Borrelia*. Parenchymatous tissues, supposedly infected by the circulatory route, contain fewer *Borrelia*. This likely reflects the fact that the organisms are more easily eliminated by the immune system in these sites. Difference in sampling technique may explain the discrepancy in results for muscle tissue between the naturally and experimentally infected dogs. *Borrelia* DNA was not detected in the kidney; however, occasionally a spirochaete has been visualized in the tubules or interstitial tissue. In one survey in Germany, approximately 15% of urine samples from dogs with cystitis and prostatitis contained *B. burgdorferi* DNA.

	Percentage positive tissues in symptomatic dogs by:			
	Culture Appel *et al.* (1993) n = 17	Culture Straubinger (2000) n = 42	PCR Chang *et al.* (1996) n = 6	PCR Hovius *et al.* (1999) n = 10
Tissue				
Skin	30	85	85	50
Lymph node	0	75	65	0
Joint capsule	25	70	95	60
Fascia	nd	70	90	nd
Muscle	50	65	100	0
Peritoneum	25	65	50	25
Pericardium	nd	80	65	nd
Heart	5	75	85	25
Meninges	nd	30	50	nd
CNS	5	nd	nd	35
Liver	0	nd	nd	60
Spleen	0	0	35	0
Kidney	5	0	0	0

nd = no data

CLINICAL SIGNS

Borreliosis in dogs (*Table 28*)

Between 1975 and 1985, novel human and canine infections were described from Old Lyme and other areas in Connecticut and from the lower Hudson Valley in New York State, USA. Dogs were described with overt lameness and swollen joints, mostly combined with fever. Although the lameness spontaneously resolved in four days, 33% of dogs relapsed. Similarities with human Lyme disease were recognized. In one dog, spirochaetes were visualized microscopically within the synoviae and identified by immunofluorescence as *B. burgdorferi*. In another canine case from the same area, *B. burgdrferi* was implicated as the cause of fever and lameness by blood culture. This lameness associated with fever was described as intermittent and shifting, with involvement of several joints.

In clinical practice, confirmation of the aetiological agent by detection of live spirochaetes is uncommon. However, in experimental and some clinical cases the spirochaete is most often detected in skin and joints, although there is only mild pathology in these tissues (**109**). More often, a presumptive diagnosis is made based on compatible clinical signs of acute malaise (fatigue, anorexia and fever) followed by recurrent lameness (stiff gait, joint swelling, arthralgia), and on the exclusion of other differential diagnoses (**110**). The period of malaise may precede lameness by days to months and its severity varies from listlessness to high fever (pyrexia occurs in 60–70% of cases).

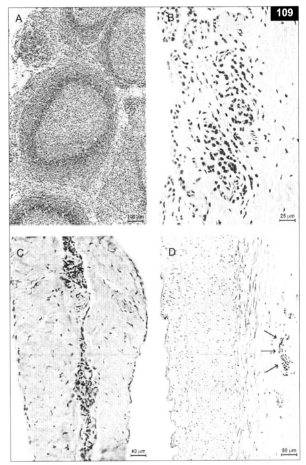

100 Histopathological lesions in borreliosis. Lesions occur in many organ systems and are characterized by an infiltration of plasma cells and lymphocytes, as seen in experimental infection. (A) Severe follicular hyperplasia of the lymph node adjacent to the location of tick bite (infection). (B) Accumulation of plasma cells in the synovial membrane of the joint near the site of a tick bite. (C) Mild non-suppurative pericarditis. A naturally infected case in the USA presented with a complete heart block, showing plasmacytic interstitial myocarditis with macrophage infiltration and focal fibre necrosis. (D) Periarteritis, visible as small cuffs of mononuclear cells around the vasa vasorum in artery walls, is frequently seen in experimental infection. (Reprinted with permission of Elsevier Science from Straubinger RK, Rao TD, Davidson E, Summers BA, Frey AB (2001) Protection against tick-transmitted Lyme disease in dogs vaccinated with a multiantigenic vaccine. *Vaccine* **20**, 181–93)

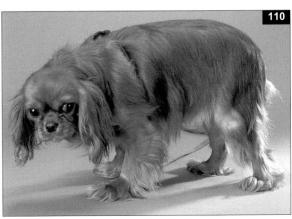

110 A four-year-old Cavalier King Charles Spaniel with a history of recurrent malaise, pyrexia, generalized musculoskeletal pain and polyarthritis. The dog is both serologically positive (rising titre) and PCR positive (blood) for *Borrelia*

Clinical signs relate not only to joint disease but also to multiple organ involvement. The skin is seldom visibly affected and the easily recognizable erythema migrans (EM) lesion seen in human infections does not occur in dogs. There is some evidence suggesting that mild localized excoriation and alopecia may be associated with infection, but this is difficult to distinguish from acute dermatitis initiated by the tick bite. Cardiac involvement is rarely observed clinically but is well described pathologically. Hepatic disease suggested by hepatomegaly and elevation of serum liver enzymes has been reported. In Europe, a non-specific reactive hepatitis has been observed on liver biopsy, and this is associated with detectable levels of *B. garinii* DNA in liver tissue. Renal involvement occurs frequently and may be an immunopathological sequela to the infection, since borreliae are only occasionally detected in the kidney tissues (*Table 28*). Severe renal disease with membranoproliferative glomerulonephritis ('canine Lyme nephritis') has been reported in the USA, most frequently in Golden and Labrador Retrievers. This is characterized by azotaemia, haematuria and urinary casts, with progression to irreversible uraemia. In Europe, a familial glomerulopathy preceded by fever and lameness has been described in Bernese Mountain Dogs, with a similar clinical and pathological progression.

Involvement of the peripheral nervous system in canine borreliosis has been described and is manifested by loss of proprioception, hyperaesthesia, posterior paresis or unilateral facial paralysis. Central nervous system involvement may manifest as aggression and epilepsy. Generally, mild to severe inflammatory infiltrates are seen in the nervous system and the spirochaete is detected in 30–50% of clinical cases in the meninges or CSF (*Table 28*).

Borreliosis in cats

Reports of naturally occurring feline borreliosis are rare. In one UK study, positive *Borrelia* serology was not associated with clinical signs of lameness or fever, and clinical signs seen in seropositive cats were not attributable to the spirochaete. Most seropositive cats had antibodies against OspA, as occurs in sera from convalescent young dogs, further suggesting that cats clear the infection without developing clinical signs. Experimentally infected cats exhibited recurrent lymphocytosis and eosinophilia every 2–3 months, with concurrent hyperplasia of lymphoid tissue. Despite minimal clinical signs (a minority of cats exhibited slight lameness), infected cats had histopathological lesions that paralleled those of natural canine infection. Lesions included perivascular lymphocytic infiltration of joint capsules, cerebrum, meninges, kidney and liver, and mild multifocal pneumonia.

DIAGNOSIS

Clinical diagnosis

The clinical signs described above are not pathognomonic and dogs lack a clinical marker like EM in humans. Consequently, making a definitive diagnosis based on clinical signs alone is not possible. As the onset of *Borrelia*-associated lameness often occurs after the period of fever and malaise, it may be difficult to make a diagnosis on the basis of a single consultation. In addition, the specific antibody response may reduce antigen load, thus modifying the expression of clinical signs. *Borrelia* species or strain variation, or co-infection with other arthropod-borne pathogens, may also alter clinical presentation.

A presumptive diagnosis of borreliosis is based on a history of tick exposure, compatible clinical signs, including a history of recurrence, and exclusion of other causes of non-degenerative arthropathy and fever of unknown origin. In particular, other immune-mediated causes of fever and shifting limb lameness should be considered. A definitive diagnosis of borreliosis always requires the addition of appropriate serological, molecular or microbiological tests.

Laboratory detection of exposure and disease

Confirmation of the clinical diagnosis of borreliosis is difficult and requires correlation and realistic interpretation of multiple laboratory investigations. Results from a European reference laboratory show that only 4.3% of sera from dogs clinically diagnosed as having borreliosis have significantly high *Borrelia* antibody titres. However, very high titres were found in 24.6% of sera from Bernese Mountain Dogs with suspected borreliosis (**111**). These data correlate with the recognized predisposition of this breed to clinical disease. It is also evident that disease due to *Borrelia* infection would be overdiagnosed if based on positive serological results alone.

Serology and western blotting

A single IgG antibody test (IFA or ELISA) is insufficient to support a diagnosis of active borreliosis, as persistent antibody production occurs in asymptomatic dogs. In addition, as disease does not often develop after the first infection, an increase in specific IgM antibodies is limited as a marker for active infection. Although a fourfold rising IgG titre in paired samples is strongly supportive of active *Borrelia* infection as the cause of disease, the time involved in confirming the diagnosis may make this impractical. As symptomatic dogs with borreliosis have significantly higher *Borrelia*-specific IgG antibody titres than asymptomatic dogs (**112**), very high titres are useful in supporting a diagnosis of clinical borreliosis, which should be confirmed using western blotting, PCR or culture (**113**). However, when low to moderate *Borrelia* titres are encountered, consideration of other differential diagnoses is recommended.

111 Frequency distribution of the antibody titres of sera from dogs with a putative clinical diagnosis of borreliosis submitted to the referral laboratory of Utrecht University, the Netherlands. Around 4% of these dogs have a very high IgG antibody titre in whole cell ELISA (log reciprocal 8 and higher) and may thus be suspected of having borreliosis. Referral sera from Bernese Mountain Dogs have an even greater fraction (around 25%) of very high titres and this breed may have high susceptibility for borreliosis. The data would suggest that borreliosis is clinically overdiagnosed.

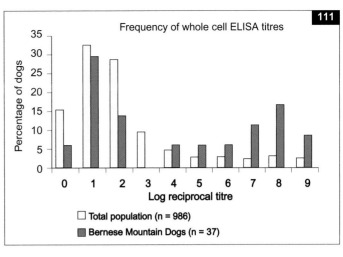

111

Frequency of whole cell ELISA titres

□ Total population (n = 986)
■ Bernese Mountain Dogs (n = 37)

112 Boxplots of IgG antibody titres of symptomatic and asymptomatic dogs. Studies from Kornblatt *et al.* 1985, Connecticut, USA and Hovius *et al.* 2000, The Netherlands, Europe are compared. Values in the latter study are more condensed because they are the highest titres measured during a five-year period. Values from the USA are from a cross-sectional study. Statistically, symptomatic dogs have higher titres; however, around 20% of asymptomatic dogs may have a high titre (of log reciprocal titre 8 = 1/2560). In the practical situation, when this high titre is encountered, it is advisable to perform a second test for confirmation of the putative diagnosis.

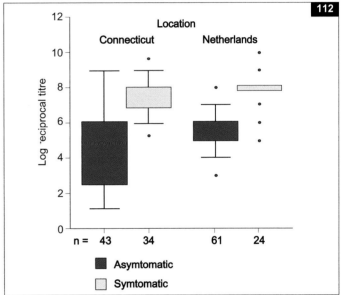

112

■ Asymtomatic
□ Symtomatic

113 (A) Antibody dynamics of a Golden Retriever acutely developing fever and lameness in its fourth year in association with a steep rising titre in whole cell ELISA. The dog was treated with antibiotics and disease resolved, while the titre declined and remained low. (B) Western blots were performed before, during and after disease. The p41 and p39 bands were weakly present, indicating asymptomatic infection before disease. More bands become apparent during disease and p30 and p28 are particularly visible against the B31 strain of *B. burgdorferi sensu stricto*. In the convalescent state, OspA antibodies are detected.

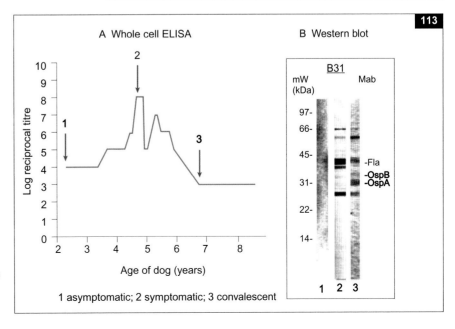

113

1 asymptomatic; 2 symptomatic; 3 convalescent

Molecular diagnosis

The presence of *Borrelia* DNA in tissue or body fluids (blood, joint fluid, CSF) can be determined by PCR analysis using *Borrelia* genes encoding molecules such as flagellin or OspA, or the intergenic spacer region of ribosomal 5S and 23S RNA, as targets. The species of *Borrelia* involved can be determined by species-specific PCR, DNA sequencing and/or hybridization of amplicons, using species-specific oligonucleotide probes. PCR positivity has been correlated with the presence of clinical symptoms; however, because of its sensitivity, PCR positivity in dogs in highly endemic areas may reflect the high risk of exposure to infected ticks, rather than clinically significant infection. Interpretation of PCR data will be greatly facilitated by the increasing availability of quantitative PCR to determine and monitor infectious load. The presence of *Borrelia* DNA in tissue or fluid samples from dogs more than 90 days after a tick bite (i.e. in the winter months in Europe) confirms persistent infection and if accompanied by disease, is highly supportive of chronic borreliosis.

Bacterial culture

Isolation of *Borrelia burgdorferi* by culture is difficult and is only successful by employing Barbour–Stoenner–Kelly (BSK) liquid medium. The medium should be inspected weekly for two months for the presence of spirochaetes by dark-field microscopy. After isolation, *Borrelia* are readily grown and multiply rapidly after passage. Bacterial culture of skin biopsies taken from the edge of an EM lesion in infected humans is a highly sensitive method for confirming the presence of *Borrelia*, and is used as the 'gold standard' for diagnosis. Blood is not considered the sample of choice since *Borrelia burgdorferi* migration is seldom haematogenous. Although spirochaetes were recovered by culture in 100% of skin biopsy samples taken two weeks after experimental infection of dogs, a positive skin culture of naturally infected dogs was only seldom achieved.

Organisms in skin and joint tissue samples from healthy dogs in endemic areas are rarely detected but when found they are considered to be the result of transient infection episodes due to current natural exposure. Consequently, as for conventional molecular diagnosis, a positive culture under these conditions does not necessarily confirm *Borrelia* as the cause of disease. However, a positive culture in a symptomatic dog that has not been exposed to infected ticks for several months confirms the presence of active infection and would strongly support the diagnosis of borreliosis.

TREATMENT AND CONTROL

Antibiotic therapy

Recovery from infection is ultimately dependent on activation of specific cell-mediated immunity and production of antibodies against OspA protecting against reinfection (**113**). Disease can be induced if immunity is disrupted by administration of high-dose corticosteroids. The effect of antibiotic therapy on the course of infection is difficult to evaluate clinically, as the episodes of lameness and fever usually resolve spontaneously after four days without treatment. However, antibiotics may help to eradicate infection if administered at the optimum time post infection. In experimentally infected dogs, administration of antibiotics prior to development of an appropriate immune response resulted in failure to clear spirochaete infection. Antibiotic therapy is most effective when administered during the first disease episode, when antibody titre is high but before the organism sequestrates. The spirochaete load is greatly reduced after antibiotic treatment and *Borrelia*-specific antibody declines in parallel. However, in a minority of experimentally and naturally infected dogs with chronic infection, spirochaetes can still be detected by PCR 500 days after treatment. It is hypothesized that spirochaetes evade antibiotic therapy within tissue cysts or 'privileged sites', such as fibroblasts.

Doxycycline (10 mg/kg p/o q12h for 28 days) is the antibiotic of choice for borreliosis because of its intracellular penetration and concurrent effects on co-infecting *Anaplasma* and *Ehrlichia* species. High-dose amoxycillin (20 mg/kg p/o q8h for 28 days) may be a better choice in very young animals because of the effects of tetracyclines on enamel formation.

Vaccination

A whole cell American strain (B31) bacterin vaccine is licensed and widely used in the northeastern USA. In a large field efficacy study using this vaccine, the incidence of borreliosis was 1% in the vaccinated group and 4.7% in non-vaccinated dogs. No adverse effects of vaccination, even on dogs previously diagnosed and recovered from borreliosis, were noted. It is estimated that around 75% of dogs in northeastern USA have been vaccinated and it has been suggested that the prevalence of canine Lyme arthritis has decreased as a consequence. The antibody response of vaccinated dogs is restricted to OspA and OspB, the 31 and 34 kDa proteins. The vaccinal antibodies are bactericidal and prevent reinfection by killing the spirochaetes in the gut of the fed tick by complement dependent activity. Active immunization with recombinant OspA renders the same protection against reinfection but only against homologous strains of *Borrelia*. Vaccination with bacterin has the advantage of eliciting higher antibody levels; however, it requires revaccination more than once a year to maintain adequate protection, after an initial course of two vaccinations three weeks apart. Mixtures of sonicated strains may confer broad enough protection in areas where different *Borrelia* strains and species occur. Recombinant OspC vaccines have not been licensed but have been shown to protect gerbils and mice from infection by inhibiting the colonization of the tick salivary gland and thus blocking transmission to the vertebrate host. It is feasible that a vaccine combining invasive OspC strains may protect against chronic infection.

Prevention

Dogs with naturally occurring borreliosis generally have a history of severe tick infestation and, in experimental infections, only dogs with high infectious loads develop fever and lameness. Consequently, prevention of heavy tick infestations by regular use of long-acting topical acaricides such as amitraz, fipronil or synthetic pyrethroids is key to prevention of disease. In addition, removing ticks within two days of attachment, before spirochaetes reach the tick salivary glands, will minimize transmission and lower infectious load. Avoidance of areas known to have a high density of ticks should be considered. The chance of acquiring pathogenic strains is also decreased with aggressive tick prevention. It is probable that owner awareness and widespread use of effective acaricides has played a role in decreasing the prevalence of canine borreliosis in the last decade.

PUBLIC HEALTH SIGNIFICANCE

Borreliosis in humans is a serious and debilitating disease with high morbidity in endemic areas. Clinical signs relate to the skin, neurological and/or musculoskeletal systems, depending on the *Borrelia* species involved. Erythema migrans typically develops within three months of an infected tick bite. This expanding rash was first described in 1910, and is now thought to indicate intradermal multiplication of spirochaetes, which disperse through the skin from the point of inoculation. All three *Borrelia* species pathogenic for man can be easily cultured or detected by PCR from these lesions. The presence of IgM antibodies confirms the diagnosis in this initial stage of human borreliosis. The second phase is marked by dissemination to multiple organ systems. In Europe, neurological disease is a more common presenting complaint than chronic arthritis. This is due to the high infection rate of European ticks with *B. garinii* and its tropism for the neurological system. Although *B. garinii* is the major species involved in neuroborreliosis, *B. afzelii* and *B. burgdorferi sensu stricto* are also isolated to a lesser extent and co-infections involving all three can occur. *B. afzelii* is almost exclusively isolated from the skin of chronically infected human patients with acrodermatitis chronica atrophicans (ACA). Although arthritis is the main symptom of *B. burgdorferi sensu stricto* infection, this species is isolated from periarticular tissues, rarely from synovial fluid.

Serological surveillance of dogs in an area endemic for borreliosis may provide information on the risk for human infection. In this respect, dogs function as sentinels. Pet dogs and cats are 'accidental hosts' for *Borrelia* and do not interface to a major degree with sylvatic wildlife cycles of *Borrelia* infection. Consequently, they pose no direct threat to human beings. However, dogs and cats may carry infected ticks into the peri-domestic environment, where there is a small risk that an infected unattached tick may be dislodged. It is unlikely that this would represent any more of a risk than exposure to infected nymphs derived from small rodents or deer with access to the garden. There is anecdotal evidence of direct transfer of infected ticks from animals to humans but no reports of disease transmission. There are no reports of humans becoming infected by dog bodily fluids, although dog urine may contain borreliae.

Precautions should be taken when removing ticks attached to dogs or cats to prevent the possibility of exposure to borreliae released from crushed tick salivary glands, which might infect small wounds on the hand, although this has never been documented. In contrast to dogs, humans may develop disease following a single tick bite, and thus should also take precautions such as wearing protective clothing when entering areas of high tick density.

10 Bartonellosis
Richard Birtles

BACKGROUND, AETIOLOGY AND EPIDEMIOLOGY

Bartonellosis is the generic name given to a wide range of infections caused by members of the genus *Bartonella*, a group of fastidious, facultatively intracellular gram-negative bacteria that are most closely related to the *Brucella* genus and members of the plant-associated taxa *Agrobacterium* and *Rhizobium*.

To date, twenty taxa have been described in association with a wide range of mammalian hosts (*Table 29*). Although not proven for all species, a general natural cycle for *Bartonella* species involves a mammalian maintenance host species, in which infection is usually chronic and asymptomatic, and a haematophagous arthropod vector that transmits infection between maintenance hosts. However, outside this cycle the occurrence of infections in non-maintenance hosts following accidental exposure to the bacteria has long been recognized. Although little is known about the relative ease with which *Bartonella* species are able to infect accidental hosts, once established, infections can lead to overt clinical manifestations, ranging from mild and self-limiting to life threatening disease. However, bartonellae may not just be opportunistic pathogens. The results of recent studies investigating the effects of parasitism on maintenance hosts have suggested that these infections too may well be detrimental to host well-being.

The nature of bartonellosis in cats is currently considered different from that in dogs. Cats are recognized as maintenance hosts for *Bartonella henselae*, the species most often implicated in human infections in the USA and Europe, and they are also likely maintenance hosts for two other species, *B. clarridgeiae* and *B. koehlerae*. To date there has been no direct demonstration of naturally occurring disease in cats caused by *B. henselae*. However, there is experimental evidence that in certain circumstances *B. henselae* infection can provoke clinical manifestations, and there is increasing speculation about the role of *B. henselae* as a cause or co-factor in chronic diseases of cats. In contrast, domestic dogs have not been clearly implicated as maintenance hosts for any *Bartonella* species, although the possibility that they may fulfil such a role cannot be ruled out. Dogs are known to be prone to chronic infections by *Bartonella vinsonii* subspecies *berkhoffii* that may be asymptomatic or may provoke overt disease. However, whether such infections are transmissible and, therefore, whether dogs serve as truly competent reservoirs, is unknown.

Arthropods as vectors of *Bartonella* species

Although the role of arthropods as vectors for *Bartonella* species is widely accepted, there is very limited evidence relating to transmission of this bacterium. Experimental transmission of *B. henselae* has been achieved by the transfer of cat fleas (*Ctenocephalides felis*) (**114**) from bacteraemic cats to specific pathogen-free (SPF) cats. Bartonellae have also been observed in the midgut of infected fleas, and they can be cultured from infected flea faeces for up to nine days post feeding. Furthermore, the intradermal inoculation of SPF cats with flea faeces has been shown to induce bacteraemia. Thus, it appears that the transmission of *B. henselae* between cats involves the uptake of infected blood by fleas, followed by multiplication of bacteria in the flea midgut, then excretion and persistence in flea faeces, and finally infection of a new host by the cutaneous inoculation of infected faeces via a scratch or abrasion.

Although experimental studies into the transmission of *B. vinsonii* subspecies *berkhoffii* have yet to be reported, epidemiological evidence suggests that ticks may be involved in this process. Evaluation of the risk factors associated with exposure to this species identified that seropositive dogs were 14 times more likely to have a history of heavy tick exposure than control animals. In addition, there appears to be a high frequency of co-infections between *B. vinsonii* subspecies *berkhoffii* and other tick-borne pathogens. Finally, surveys of questing ixodid ticks (**115**) in the USA and Europe using PCR-based methods have yielded gene sequences that are very similar to several *Bartonella* species, including some for which other arthropods have been established as vectors.

Table 29 Identity of currently recognised *Bartonella* species and details of their likely maintenance host species.

Bartonella taxon	Maintenance host	Cat/dog association
B. alsatica	Rabbit	✗
B. bacilliformis	Man	✗
B. birtlesii	Small woodland mammals	✗
B. bovis	Cow	✗
B. capreoli	Roe deer	✗
B. clarridgeiae	Cat	✓
B. doshiae	Small woodland mammals	✗
B. elizabethae	Rat	✓
B. grahamii	Small woodland mammals	✗
B. henselae	Cat	✓
B. koehlerae	Cat	✓
B. peromysci	White-footed mouse	✗
B. quintana	Man	✗
B. talpae	Mole	✗
B. taylorii	Small woodland mammals	✗
B. tribocorum	Rat	✗
B. schoenbuchii	Roe deer	✗
B. vinsonii subspecies *arupensis*	Small woodland mammals	✗
B. vinsonii subspecies *berkhoffii*	Coyote	✓
B. vinsonii subspecies *vinsonii*	Small woodland mammals	✗

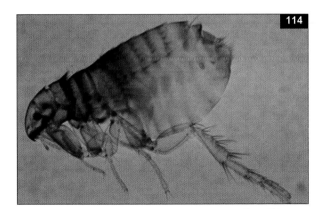

114 Photograph of *Ctenocephalides felis*, the cat flea. (Photo courtesy Merial Animal Health UK)

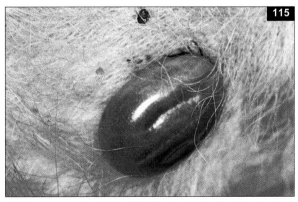

115 An engorged adult ixodid tick attached to the skin of a dog.

Bartonella henselae and *Bartonella clarridgeiae* infection of domestic cats

The role of cats as reservoir hosts for *B. henselae* and *B. clarridgeiae* has been established on the basis of extensive surveys of domestic cat populations and experimental studies of laboratory animals. *Table 30* summarizes these surveys, which have been carried out in over 20 countries and have included more than 7,000 animals. Overall, these data indicate that, worldwide, 15% of cats tested have ongoing infection and 27% of animals have evidence of past infection.

Significant differences in the prevalence of *B. henselae* infection among subsets of the cat population have been reported, leading to the recognition of a number of predisposing factors. Risk factors associated with bacteraemia include flea infestation, young age and being stray or housed in cat shelters. Among pet cats, risk factors include ownership for less than six months, adoption from a shelter/found as a stray and cohabitation with one or more cats. It has also been suggested that the prevalence of infection/exposure is inversely related to latitude. The seroprevalence of *B. henselae* is higher in cat populations living in the southern USA than in those living in the north, and recent surveys of cats in central and northern Scandinavia have found little evidence of *B. henselae* infections. This correlation may be related to warmer, more humid regions favouring *Ct. felis* infestation, but may also reflect differences in the age profile or numbers of stray/feral cats in local populations.

Feline *B. clarridgeiae* infections appear to be less common than those due to *B. henselae*. Less than half the surveys that encountered *B. henselae* also encountered *B. clarridgeiae*, and when both species were encountered, the prevalence of *B. henselae* was always the greater, with over 80% of culture-positive cats yielding *B. henselae* and only about 25% yielding *B. clarridgeiae*. However, as currently used sampling methods have been optimized for the recovery of *B. henselae*, the recovery of *B. clarridgeiae* may be compromised. The geographical distribution of *B. clarridgeiae* may also be more limited than that of *B. henselae*. The species is rarely encountered in the USA but appears more common in Europe and the Far East. Within Europe, the species is relatively widely distributed but may be absent from the UK and Scandinavia.

Table 30 National estimates of prevalence of infection and exposure among domestic cats.

Country	Year of survey(s)	Sample source	Prevalence of infection	Prevalence of exposure	Species identified*
Australia	1996	H, S	27/77, 35%	NT	BH
Austria	1995		NT	32/96, 33%	
Czech Republic	2003	H, S	5/61, 8%	NT	BH
Denmark	2002	H, S	21/93, 23%	42/92, 46%	BH
Egypt	1995		NT	8/42, 19%	
France	1995, 1997, 2001	H, S	129/594, 22%	202/500, 40%	BH, BC
Germany	1997, 1999, 2001	H, S	33/293, 11%	107/713, 15%	BH, BC
Indonesia	1999	H, S	9/14, 64%	40/74, 54%	BH, BC
Israel	1996		NT	45/114, 39%	
Italy	2002 × 2	H, S	24/264, 9%	98/427, 23%	BH
Japan	1995, 1996, 1998, 2000, 2003	H, S	181/2170, 8%	73/670, 11%	BH, BC
Netherlands	1997	H, S	25/113, 22%	85/163, 52%	BH, BC
New Zealand	1997		8/48, 17%	NT	BH
Norway	2002	H, S	0/100, 0%	1/100, 1%	
Philippines	1999		19/31, 61%	73/107, 68%	BH, BC
Portugal	1995		NT	2/14, 14%	
Singapore	1999		NT	38/80, 47%	
South Africa	1996, 1999	H, S	1/31, 3%	11/52, 21%	BH
Sweden	2002, 2003		1/100, 1%	73/292, 25%	BH
Switzerland	1997	H, S	NT	61/728, 8%	
Thailand	2001		76/275, 28%	NT	BH, BC
UK	2000, 2002	H, S	34/360, 9%	61/148, 41%	BH
USA	1994 × 2, 1995 × 4, 1996, 1998	H, S	128/323, 40%	912/2910, 31%	BH, BC
Zimbabwe	1996	H, S	NT	28/119, 24%	

* by culture-based assessment only
H = cats residing within a household; S = feral, stray or shelter-living cats; NT = not tested; BH = *Bartonella henselae*; BC = *Bartonella clarridgeiae*.

B. vinsonii subspecies berkhoffii infection of dogs

The assumption that *B. vinsonii* subspecies *berkhoffii* is always pathogenic in dogs is no longer valid. Despite good evidence that dogs are frequently exposed to *B. vinsonii* subspecies *berkhoffii*, reports of overt illness due to the species are still uncommon. Although a recent USA survey found 162 of 1,872 working dogs (9%) were seropositive for *B. vinsonii* subspecies *berkhoffii*, less than ten confirmed clinical case reports have been published. Furthermore, the species has been shown to persist subclinically for 16 months in the blood of an apparently healthy dog.

The recent demonstration of coyotes (*Canis latrans*) as a major reservoir for *B. vinsonii* subspecies *berkhoffii* has gone some way to clarifying the natural cycle of the species in the USA.

B. henselae, B. clarridgeiae and B. elizabethae infection of dogs

In many parts of the world dogs are as prone to infestation with the cat flea as cats themselves, so it is surprising that *B. henselae* infections of dogs, either clinical or subclinical, appear to be rare. A culture-based survey in the UK failed to recover a single isolate of any *Bartonella* species from over 250 dogs tested. Serosurveys have yielded some indications of infection in apparently healthy dogs, although the accuracy of a serological approach as a species-specific indicator of *Bartonella* infection is debatable. However, intriguingly, the recent unexpected detection of *B. henselae* in the peripheral blood of three dogs presenting with chronic illnesses has provoked the suggestion that dogs may act as a reservoir for the species. Interestingly, DNA derived from (rodent-reservoired) *Bartonella elizabethae* was detected in the peripheral blood of a fourth dog presented as part of the series described above, implicating this species as a canine pathogen for the first time.

There is some circumstantial evidence that dogs can transmit *B. henselae* and *B. clarridgeiae*. Reports from Japan and Israel have suggested that human cases of *B. henselae* infection may result from contact with dogs, possibly acting as vehicles for infected fleas.

Molecular epidemiology of *Bartonella* species associated with cats and dogs

Delineation of *B. henselae* isolates into one of two genogroups on the basis of differences in 16S ribosomal RNA gene sequences has long been recognized, and descriptions of isolates as type I and type II are commonplace. However, the distribution of these two types among isolates does not appear to be entirely congruent with lineages allocated using a multilocus sequence typing (MLST) approach to assess the *B. henselae* population structure. It therefore appears that distinguishing strains solely on a type I/type II basis is not a sensitive indicator of clonal divisions within the species. The population structure proposed by MLST is supported by other means of assessing inter-strain genetic relatedness, including pulsed field gel electrophoresis (PFGE).

From a molecular epidemiological perspective, several highly variable genomic loci have been identified including the 16S/23S rRNA intergenic spacer region, *groEL*, and *pap31*. PFGE (**116**), together with other pan-genomic sampling methods such as amplified fragment length polymorphism analysis, enterobacterial repetitive intergenic consensus (ERIC)-PCR and arbitrarily primed-PCR, has also been used to delineate *B. henselae* isolates. Although the majority of these investigations have been carried out on a small panel of isolates, a recent more substantial PFGE-based survey showed good correlation between the strain genotype and its geographical origin, with American and Japanese strains appearing to form discrete clusters.

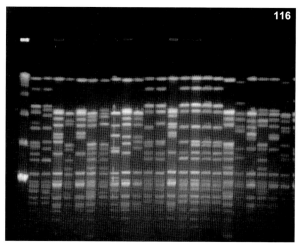

116 Macrorestriction analysis of *B. henselae* isolates by pulsed field gel electrophoretic resolution of *Sma*I digested genomic DNA. Lane 1 contains a size marker and lanes 2–29 contain DNA profiles obtained from 28 different *B. henselae* isolates obtained from cats in the UK. Variation in the profiles demonstrates the genetic variability within the species. (Picture courtesy Dr M Arvand, University of Rostock, Germany)

PATHOGENESIS

B. henselae infection in cats

Experimental infections have demonstrated that cats are prone to protracted bacteraemia of at least eight weeks, during which time the bacteria associate with, then (probably) invade, erythrocytes. The concentration of bacteria in blood rises rapidly to reach a peak within one week of inoculation, after which it gradually subsides. Although in most experiments this resulted in disappearance of bacteraemia after about three months, in some animals infection was more protracted and in others, recurrent periods of bacteraemia were observed (**117**).

Cats elicit a strong humoral response against inoculated bartonellae. Significant titres of IgG and IgM can be detected in animals within two weeks of inoculation and antibodies persist for several months. However, the evolution of immunoglobulin titres varies between individuals (**118**). Western blot analysis has allowed the identification of at least 24 *Bartonella*-specific antigens recognized by experimentally infected cats, with the kinetics of antibody appearance during infection varying with individual antigens. A large-scale survey of naturally infected cats has demonstrated that the spectrum of *B. henselae* immunogenic antigens varies between individual animals, but that a subset of the antigens recognized by experimentally infected cats are consistently encountered.

There is conflicting evidence regarding the role played by the humoral response in the abrogation of *B. henselae* bacteraemia. Experimental infection of B-cell deficient mice has demonstrated that the cessation of bacteraemia due to *Bartonella grahamii* (a species associated with woodland rodents) is antibody-mediated, as persistent bacteraemia was converted to a transient course by transfer of immune serum. However, infected cats with or without serum IgG antibodies to *B. henselae* may become blood-culture negative simultaneously, suggesting that IgG is not required to clear bacteraemia. There is no doubt that infected cats are prone to recurrent *B. henselae* bacteraemia despite the presence of circulating antibodies. However, as yet there is no evidence for the emergence of antigenic variants to explain this phenomenon, and the potential for intracellular survival of *Bartonella* in cells other than erythrocytes has not been fully investigated.

There has been very little study of the *Bartonella*-specific cell-mediated immune response. Positive cutaneous delayed hypersensitivity reactions in cats following exposure and challenge with live *B. henselae* have been reported. However, experimentally infected cats failed to make a similar response following intradermal administration of the cat scratch disease (CSD) antigen that is comprised of heat-treated pus collected from the lymph nodes of human CSD patients. The nature of the *Bartonella*-specific *in vitro* lymphocyte proliferative response has also been examined.

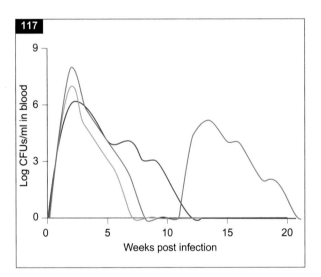

117 Examples of different types of bacteraemias detected in cats experimentally infected with *B. henselae*. The green curve represents the most commonly observed, shortest infections; the blue curve represents a more protracted infection; whereas the red curve represents recurrent bacteraemia.

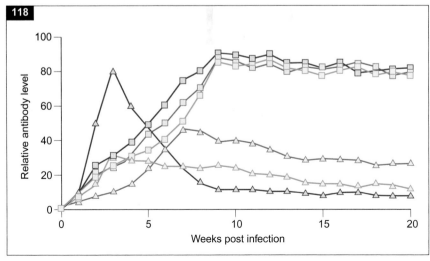

118 Examples of different types of antibody kinetics in cats experimentally infected with *B. henselae*. The relative antibody levels for IgM (Δ) and IgG (□) are shown. Type 1 (blue curves) involves an acute, strong but short-lived IgM peak, followed by a strong and protracted IgG response. Type 2 (red curves) involves a far weaker and delayed IgM response, closely followed by a strong and protracted IgG response. Type 3 (green curves) involves an acute but relatively weak IgM response, followed by a strong and protracted IgG response.

B. clarridgeiae and B. koehlerae infection in cats

Experimental infections of SPF cats with both *B. clarridgeiae* and *B. koehlerae* resulted in a subclinical chronic bacteraemia similar to that seen with *B. henselae*. Comparison of infection kinetics indicated that cats inoculated with *B. koehlerae* have a shorter duration of bacteraemia than those inoculated with *B. clarridgeiae*, and none developed relapsing bacteraemia. All infected cats mounted a humoral response against the specific inoculum. There were no apparent differences in the course of infection between cats inoculated with blood co-infected with *B. henselae* and *B. clarridgeiae* and those inoculated with *B. henselae* alone.

B. vinsonii subspecies berkhoffii infection in dogs

Current understanding of the pathogenesis of *B. vinsonii* subspecies *berkhoffii* infection in dogs is very limited. However, a recent immunopathological study of the species in experimentally infected dogs found that despite production of substantial levels of specific antibody, *B. vinsonii* subspecies *berkhoffii* was able to establish chronic infection. This resulted in immune suppression characterized by defects in monocytic phagocytosis, decreased numbers of peripheral blood CD8+ T lymphocytes, together with phenotypic alteration of their cell surface, and an increase in CD4+ lymphocytes in the peripheral lymph nodes.

Demonstration of microscopic lesions in cardiac tissue from naturally infected dogs has been used to infer *B. vinsonii* subspecies *berkhoffii* pathogenicity. Multiple foci of myocarditis and endocarditis have been observed, leading to the suggestion that bartonellae may preferentially colonize previously damaged tissue and that once colonization is established, a progressive inflammatory response develops to the organisms.

CLINICOPATHOLOGICAL SIGNS OF FELINE BARTONELLOSIS

It is generally believed that the cost of *B. henselae* parasitism to the feline host is minimal. However, there is evidence that some strains of *B. henselae* may provoke overt clinical signs in cats, and that hosting chronic *Bartonella* infection is detrimental.

Experimental infection with B. henselae

Clinical and pathological evaluations of experimentally infected cats have yielded inconsistent results, which may reflect differences in experimental procedure between different studies. Although in most animals clinical signs were minimal and gross necropsy findings were unremarkable, histopathological findings have included inflammatory foci in the kidneys, heart, liver and spleen and in the peripheral lymph nodes. Less commonly, overt clinical signs have been described including fever, lethargy, transient anaemia, lymphadenomegaly and neurological dysfunction. Some cats experimentally infected with *B. henselae* developed delayed conception or lack of conception, or fetal involution or resorption.

Only one group of researchers has consistently reported clinical disease resulting from experimental inoculation of laboratory cats, including the development of injection site reactions followed by fever and lethargy. It was proposed that the isolate of *B. henselae* associated with the atypical clinical observations was a more 'virulent' strain, implying that the virulence of *B. henselae* in cats is strain dependent. This hypothesis has not yet been tested elsewhere.

Disease association in natural feline B. henselae infection

Disease association with naturally occurring *B. henselae* infection is difficult to determine because of its high prevalence in asymptomatic cats. In Japan, one survey demonstrated that seropositivity for *B. henselae* and feline immunodeficiency virus was significantly associated with a history of lymphadenopathy and gingivitis. Similarly, a survey of cats from the USA and the Caribbean found that seropositivity was significantly associated with fevers of unknown origin, gingivitis, stomatitis, lymphadenopathy and uveitis (**119**). In support of this final finding, a further survey in the USA demonstrated that 14% of cats suffering from uveitis, but no healthy cats, had detectable *Bartonella* antibodies in their aqueous humour. In a Swiss survey of over 700 cats, there was significant correlation between high *B. henselae* antibody titres and a range of renal and urinary tract abnormalities. Furthermore, all sick cats over seven years old in this survey were seropositive.

Individual case reports supporting these associations are almost entirely lacking. In one cat with anterior uveitis, significant ocular production of *Bartonella*-specific antibodies was demonstrated, supporting this as the aetiological agent. *B. henselae* has also been unconvincingly associated with vegetative endocarditis in two cats.

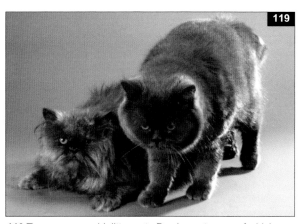

119 Two one-year-old, littermate Persian cats, one of which has a febrile syndrome with pyogranulomatous lymphadenitis. Blood from the cat was PCR positive for *B. henselae*. The histopathological appearance of a lymph node biopsy from this cat is shown in **122** and **123**.

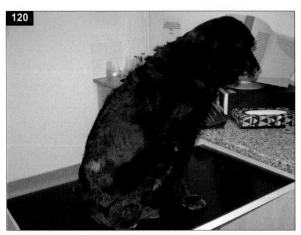
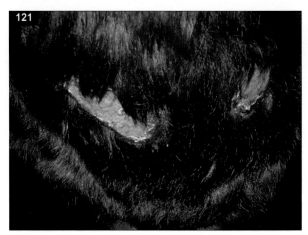

120, 121 A ten-year-old, neutered female Labrador-cross dog with a history of generalized lymphadenopathy, pyrexia, lethargy, grade III cardiac murmur and localized areas of ulceration over the gluteal region. Histopathology revealed pyogranulomatous dermatitis and necrotizing lymphadenitis, and Warthin–Starry staining of the lymph node revealed the presence of organisms consistent with *Bartonella* species. Blood from the dog was PCR positive for *Bartonella* species. The dog had been previously treated with glucocorticoids for polyarthritis.

CLINICOPATHOLOGICAL SIGNS OF CANINE BARTONELLOSIS

Most *Bartonella*-associated disease in dogs has been associated with *B. vinsonii* subspecies *berkhoffii* infection. However, as only a small number of cases have been recognized, the true spectrum of clinical manifestations induced by *Bartonella* species in dogs must be considered virtually unknown. Of the eight confirmed cases of *B. vinsonii* subspecies *berkhoffii* infection, two were asymptomatic, four presented with endocarditis and two had granulomatous disease (**120, 121**). A number of possible co-infections involving *B. vinsonii* subspecies *berkhoffii* and *Ehrlichia* species have also been reported.

Both *B. clarridgeiae* and *B. henselae* have been associated with rare clinical disease in dogs. *B. clarridgeiae* was identified in blood culture from a single fatal case of canine endocarditis. In addition, *B. clarridgeiae* DNA was detected in the deformed aortic valve and the dog was also seropositive for *Bartonella* species. *B. henselae* has been implicated as a causative agent in a case of canine peliosis hepatis following the detection of species DNA in affected hepatic tissue. Very recently, *B. henselae* has also been associated with chronic illness in three dogs. Although each animal presented with varying clinical manifestations, severe weight loss, protracted lethargy and anorexia were common to all three. All three dogs also possessed similar haematological and biochemical abnormalities that included eosinophilia, monocytosis, alterations in platelet numbers and elevated serum amylase. *B. henselae* was implicated in the pathogenesis by the detection of DNA in peripheral blood samples. The clinical relevance of these microbiological findings is difficult to infer from such a small case number, particularly given the degree of variation in clinical, haematological and biochemical abnormalities observed. Furthermore, two of the dogs had other concurrent disease. However, the fact that several features were shared among the animals, and that all responded well to appropriate antibiosis (in one case in conjunction with glucocorticoids), may support a pathogenic role for *B. henselae*.

DIAGNOSIS

Difficulties in interpreting the significance of positive blood cultures and serology, particularly in cats, necessitate the use of multiple diagnostic methods. Although isolation of a *Bartonella* species by blood culture from a non-reservoir host (e.g. *B. henselae* or *B. clarridgeiae* from an ill dog) is supportive of its role as a causative agent, diagnosis of bartonellosis is best confirmed by demonstration of bartonellae in infected tissues using histological, immunohistological or molecular methods (**122, 123**).

Histology and immunohistochemistry

The value of histopathology in the diagnosis of naturally occurring *Bartonella* infections has only really been explored in dogs. The histopathological presentation of endocarditis and myocarditis due to infection with *B. vinsonii* subspecies *berkhoffii* is quite characteristic. In one of the two reports of granulomatous disease in dogs associated with *B. vinsonii* subspecies *berkhoffii*, Warthin–Starry (WS) silver staining of tissue sections revealed the presence of clusters of rod-like organisms within and between cells. However, in the second report the stain failed to detect any organisms. A similar degree of inconsistency was apparent during diagnosis of *B. vinsonii* subspecies *berkhoffii*-associated endocarditis. In the first case report, WS and Gram staining revealed intense bacterial colonization of the margins of the infected valves, whereas in a subsequent case, no organisms were apparent. Transmission electron microscopy has also been used to demonstrate the presence of gram-negative bacteria in tissue sections (**124**).

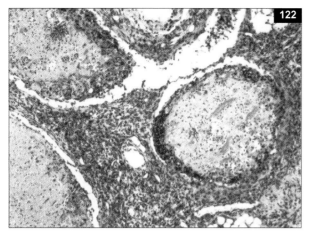

122 Section of lymph node from cat with bartonellosis. Within the medullary area there are foci of necrosis associated with mixed mononuclear cell inflammation.

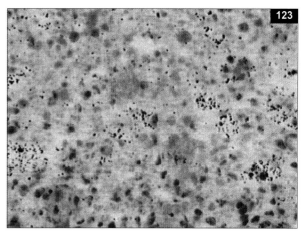

123 Section of lymph node from cat with bartonellosis stained by the Warthin–Starry method. The darkly stained aggregates are consistent with the expected appearance of *Bartonella* colonies.

124 Transmission electron microscopic image of *Bartonella henselae*. The outer surface of the bacterium is pilated. (×146,000) (Photo courtesy Dr J Iredell, University of Sydney, Australia)

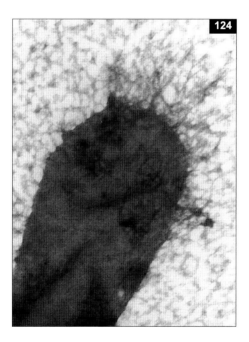

125 *B. henselae* colonies growing on blood agar eight days after the plate was inoculated with the blood of an infected cat. The plate was incubated at 35°C, in a 5% CO$_2$ atmosphere.

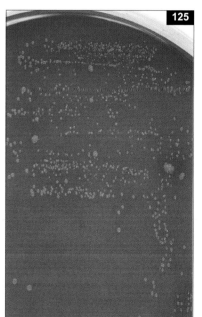

Isolation of *Bartonella* species

The recovery of bartonellae from the blood of naturally infected reservoirs is relatively straightforward, whereas their recovery from non-reservoir (accidental) hosts is extremely difficult. The cultivation of *B. henselae* and *B. clarridgeiae* from the blood of cats untreated by antibiotics is, therefore, relatively simple, requiring prolonged incubation of inoculated blood-rich agar plates at 35–37°C in a moist, 5% CO$_2$ atmosphere. Colonies of bartonellae become visible between five and 15 days and are usually small, cauliflower-like, dry and of an off-white colour (**125**), although often a 'wetter' phenotype occurs,

with colonies appearing smoother and shiny. There is some evidence to suggest that the manner in which blood samples are handled may influence the success of culture. Two procedures that enhance recovery of *B. henselae* from infected cat blood are: (1) freezing samples to –80°C for 24 hours prior to testing; and (2) collection of blood into isolator blood lysis tubes rather than EDTA tubes.

The isolation of *B. vinsonii* subspecies *berkhoffii* from coyotes has been achieved using methods similar to those described for the isolation of *B. henselae* from cats. However, using these methods, the recovery of isolates from the tissues of infected dogs appears to be far less efficient.

Serological methods

Detection of circulating antibodies to *Bartonella* species has been performed using several different assay formats including IFATs, ELISAs and western blotting. Antigens for use in these assays are usually whole bacteria that have been cultivated either on agar plates or, more often, in association with eukaryotic cell cultures. Serology is most commonly performed on serum/plasma samples but most body fluid samples, including aqueous humour, can be used.

In cats, serum IgG is very persistent, which limits the diagnostic usefulness of elevated antibody levels as an indicator of ongoing infection. Investigation of the relationship between infection status and seropositivity, using a convenience sample of about 200 cats in the USA, revealed that antibody titres were higher in bacteraemic cats than in non-bacteraemic cats, and that younger age and seropositivity to *B. henselae* were associated with bacteraemia. However, as expected, the estimated positive predictive value of seropositivity as an indicator of bacteraemia was found to be less than 50%, underlining the limited value of the assay.

In the canine cases reported to date for which serological data are available, significant antibody levels were detected. However, as several surveys have demonstrated significant antibody titres in apparently healthy dogs, the predictive value of serology for diagnosing clinical disease due to *B. vinsonii* subspecies *berkhoffii* is likely to be limited.

The interpretation of *Bartonella* serological results has also been compromised by presumed cross-reactivity. Certainly there is marked cross-reaction among *Bartonella* species, although not with antigens derived from close relatives of the Bartonellaceae (*Brucella canis*, *Ehrlichia canis* and *Rickettsia rickettsii*). However, cross-reactivity between *Bartonella* antigens and the antisera of dogs with molecular evidence of infection due to non-*Bartonella* α-subgroup Proteobacteria has been reported.

Molecular methods

A number of molecular methodologies have been developed for the diagnosis of human *Bartonella* infections and some have been successfully applied to veterinary medicine. PCR-based methods have been described, targeting a range of DNA fragments. However, the sensitivity of these methods for the detection of *Bartonella* DNA in infected blood appears limited and in several comparative surveys they have not performed as well as culture. Nonetheless, as tools for the detection of *Bartonella* DNA in the tissues of diseased animals, PCR-based methods have proven useful additions to histological and serological methods. Genomic targets for PCRs include fragments of the 16S rRNA-encoding gene or the 16S/23S intergenic spacer region, and the citrate synthase-encoding gene (*gltA*) (**126**).

TREATMENT AND CONTROL

Antibiotic therapy

The treatment of *B. henselae* bacteraemia in cats is problematic. Doxycycline, amoxicillin and amoxicillin/clavulanate used at higher than recommended dose rates have been reported to be successful in suppressing bacteraemia in experimental infections. However, more detailed study suggested that although enrofloxacin was more efficacious than doxycycline for the treatment of *B. henselae* or *B. clarridgeiae*, neither drug eliminated the infection in all animals, even when administered for four weeks. Data relating to the treatment of naturally infected animals are scant. However, because of the difficulty in eliminating bacteraemia, antibiotic therapy is only recommended for those cats that have confirmed *Bartonella*-associated disease or those in contact with immunosuppressed owners.

Treatment of canine endocarditis due to *B. vinsonii* subspecies *berkhoffii* is also difficult. There has been no clinical response reported to therapeutic protocols incorporating amoxicillin, enrofloxacin, cephalexin, doxycycline and amikacin in combination with diuretics and various combinations of cardiovascular drugs. Two dogs with granulomatous disease due to *B. vinsonii* subspecies *berkhoffii* appeared to respond well to antibiotics: a three-week course of enrofloxacin (12.5 mg/kg q12h) in the first case and a 30-day course of doxycycline (5.4 mg/kg q12h) in the second.

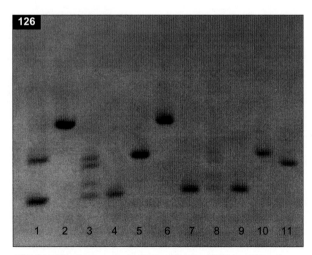

126 Amplification products derived from a PCR targeting the 16S/23S rRNA intergenic spacer region of *Bartonella* species. Different *Bartonella* species yield different sized products, as revealed by their resolution on a 3% agarose gel. Lanes 3 and 8 contain size markers.

Ectoparasite control

Ectoparasitic control should be of great prophylactic benefit in preventing transmission of *B. henselae* and *B. clarridgeiae* infection between cats. However, despite the availability and use of effective flea adulticide treatments, *Bartonella* infections remain common, even in the domestic cat populations of industrialized, affluent countries of Europe and North America. As yet no studies have been carried out examining the efficacy of different ectoparasiticides in the prevention of *B. henselae* transmission. Until proven otherwise, it is feasible that fleas introduced to ectoparasite-treated animals have the capacity to transmit infection before being affected.

ZOONOTIC POTENTIAL/PUBLIC HEALTH SIGNIFICANCE

The zoonotic potential of *B. henselae* is enormous. For example, in the UK, 4.5 million households (or more than 1 in 4) house over 7.5 million cats, of which about 10% are *B. henselae* bacteraemic. The potential threat of this reservoir is reflected in the frequency with which humans acquire *B. henselae* infections, most commonly manifesting as CSD. In the USA, about 24,000 cases of CSD are reported each year, of which about 2,000 require hospitalization. Fortunately, this syndrome is usually benign and self-limiting, manifesting as a regional lymphadenopathy and affecting mainly children and young adults (**127**). However, systemic complications may arise leading to more profound diseases. Accurate diagnosis of CSD is important as it requires differentiation from other potentially more serious causes of lymphadenitis such as abscesses, lymphoma, mycobacterial infections, toxoplasmosis and Kawasaki disease.

When first characterized in the late 1980s, *B. henselae* was specifically associated with opportunistic infections in AIDS patients. The advent of more effective prophylactic therapy for these patients has seen the incidence of these infections decline in the USA and Europe, although they are likely to remain a significant health burden in Africa and other developing parts of the world where therapies are not currently affordable. However, medical interest in zoonotic bartonellae continues today, as an increasing spectrum of syndromes among immunocompetent individuals is encountered. Perhaps of most relevance currently is the emergence of *B. henselae* in the aetiologies of ocular syndromes such as uveitis and neuroretinitis.

B. clarridgeiae has also been implicated as an agent of CSD and *B. vinsonii* subspecies *berkhoffii* has, on one occasion, been identified as the aetiological agent of endocarditis.

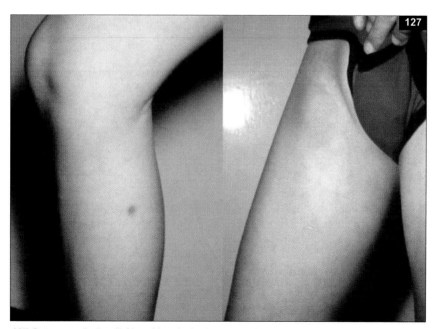

127 Cutaneous lesion (left) and inguinal adenopathy (right) in a boy following a cat scratch on his right leg. (Photo courtesy Dr C Wilkinson, Nottingham Public Health Laboratory, UK)

11 Ehrlichiosis and anaplasmosis

Shimon Harrus, Trevor Waner,
Anneli Bjöersdorff and Susan Shaw

INTRODUCTION

Until recently, three groups of intracellular bacterial organisms within the genus *Ehrlichia* (family Rickettsiaceae) were recognized as pathogenic in animals and humans. Reclassification based on phylogenetic analysis of gene sequences, including the 16S rRNA gene, has resulted in the formation of three separate genera:

- **Genus *Ehrlichia*** retains the 'type' species *Ehrlichia canis*, the cause of monocytic ehrlichiosis in dogs and possibly cats. Other species infecting dogs, primarily in the USA, include *E. chaffeensis* and *E. ewingii*.
- **Genus *Anaplasma*** now includes the 'type' species *Anaplasma phagocytophilum*, the cause of granulocytic 'ehrlichiosis' in dogs and cats, and *A. platys*, the cause of canine infectious cyclic thrombocytopenia.

- **Genus *Neorickettsia*** includes the 'type' species *Neorickettsia risticii*, the cause of Potomac horse fever in the USA. There are also species that cause canine infection and disease in the USA. Cats are susceptible to experimental infection with *N. risticii*, and serological evidence of naturally occurring infection has been reported.

Of these, organisms in the genera *Ehrlichia* and *Anaplasma* are tick-transmitted and are discussed in this chapter. The relationships of those species causing naturally occurring disease in dogs and cats to the other species in the genera are illustrated (**128**). Members of the genus *Neorickettsia* are non-arthropod transmitted.

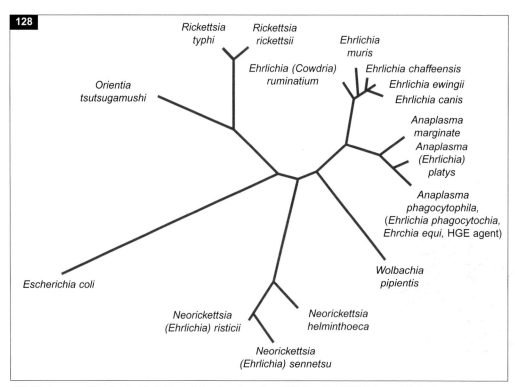

128 Phylogeny of the family Ehrlichiae. (After Dumler JS and Walker DH (2001) *Lancet Infectious Diseases* **April**, 21–28).

PART 1: *EHRLICHIA CANIS* GENOGROUP

Shimon Harrus and Trevor Waner

EHRLICHIA CANIS

Background, aetiology and epidemiology

Ehrlichia canis, the principal member of the *E. canis* genogroup (*Table 31*), is a small pleomorphic gram-negative, coccoid, obligatory intracellular bacterium. It is the aetiological agent of canine monocytic ehrlichiosis (CME), a tick-borne disease previously known as tropical canine pancytopenia. *E. canis* parasitizes circulating monocytes intracytoplasmically in clusters of organisms called morulae (**129**, **130**). It infects dogs and other members of the Canidae family. *E. canis* was first identified by Donatien and Lestoquard in Algeria in 1935 and since then CME has been recognized worldwide as an important canine disease. CME gained much attention when hundreds of American military dogs, many of which were German Shepherd Dogs, died from the disease during the Vietnam War. *E. canis* received further attention in the late 1980s, when the organism was erroneously suspected to infect humans.

Ehrlichial morulae have been detected in leucocytes of cats and seropositivity for *E. canis* has been detected in both domestic and wild cats. Recently, *E. canis* DNA has been identified in the blood of three sick cats but to date, attempts to culture *E. canis* from suspected feline cases have been unsuccessful. The potential of *E. canis* to infect cats and cause disease has yet to be determined.

Table 31 Members of the *Ehrlichia canis* genogroup infecting canines[1]: their geographic distribution, vectors, hosts and target cells.

Ehrlichial species	Geographic distribution	Primary vector	Primary host	Target cell
E. canis	Worldwide, not Australia	*Rhipicephalus sanguineus*	Canids	Monocyte, macrophage
E. ewingii	USA	*Amblyomma americanum*	Canids	Neutrophil, eosinophil
E. chaffeensis	USA	*Amblyomma americanum*	Humans	Monocyte, macrophage

[1] The **Ehrlichia canis** genogroup includes another two members: *Cowdria ruminantium,* which infects ruminants, and *E. muris,* which infects mice. These two members have not been reported naturally to infect dogs or cats.

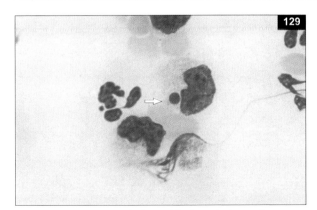

129 *Ehrlichia canis* morula (arrow) in the cytoplasm of a monocyte as visualized in a blood smear. (Giemsa stain, original magnification ×1,000)

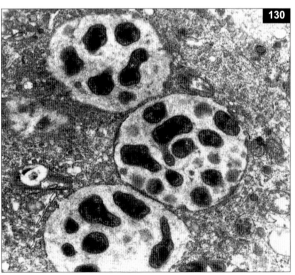

130 Morulae consisting of many *Ehrlichia canis* organisms in the cytoplasm of tissue culture cells (DH82 macrophages) as visualized by electron microscopy. (Original magnification ×20,000)

E. canis is transmitted by *Rhipicephalus sanguineus* (the brown dog tick) (**131**). Experimentally, it has also been transmitted by *Dermacentor variabilis* (the American dog tick). Transmission in the tick occurs transstadially but not transovarially. Larvae and nymphs become infected while feeding on rickettsaemic dogs and transmit the infection to the host after moulting to nymphs and adults, respectively. Throughout feeding, ticks inject *E. canis*-contaminated salivary gland secretions into the feeding site. Adult ticks have been shown to transmit infection 155 days after becoming infected. This phenomenon allows ticks to overwinter and infect hosts in the following spring. The occurrence and geographical distribution of CME are related to the distribution and biology of its vector. *R. sanguineus* ticks are abundant during the warm season; therefore, most acute cases of CME occur during this period. As *R. sanguineus* ticks are cosmopolitan, the disease has a worldwide distribution (Asia, Europe, Africa and America). Dogs living in endemic regions and those travelling to endemic areas should be considered potential candidates for infection. Infection with *E. canis* may also occur through infected blood transfusions, therefore screening of blood donors is extremely important.

Pathogenesis

The incubation period of CME is 8–20 days. During this period, ehrlichial organisms enter the bloodstream and lymphatics and localize in macrophages, mainly in the spleen and liver, where they replicate by binary fission. From there, infected macrophages disseminate the infection to other organ systems. It is likely that the mechanism by which ehrlichiae survive and multiply in the infected cell relies on their ability to inhibit phagosome-lysosome fusion. Doxycycline has been shown to restore this function in cells infected with *N. risticii* and *N. sennetsu*. The incubation period is followed consecutively by an acute, a subclinical and a chronic phase:

- The acute phase may last 1–4 weeks; most dogs recover in this phase provided there is adequate treatment.
- Untreated dogs and those treated inappropriately may enter the subclinical phase of the disease. Dogs in this phase may remain persistent carriers of *E. canis* for months or years. It has been proposed that persistent infection is facilitated by repeated recombination of the outer membrane protein genes of the organism, thus allowing immune evasion. The spleen plays a major role in the pathogenesis of the disease and the persistence of *E. canis* infection, and some studies suggest that splenic macrophages harbour the rickettsiae during the carrier phase.
- Some persistently infected dogs may recover spontaneously; however, others subsequently develop the chronic severe form of the disease. Not all dogs develop the chronic phase of CME, and factors leading to the development of this phase remain unclear. The prognosis at this stage is grave, and death may occur as a consequence of haemorrhage and/or secondary infection.

Immunological mechanisms appear to be involved in the pathogenesis of the disease. Positive Coombs and autoagglutination tests indicate that infection induces the production of antibodies that bind to the membrane of erythrocytes. Whether these are true autoantibodies (red cell antigen-specific) has not been determined. The demonstration of platelet-bound antibodies in infected animals suggests that these play a role in the pathogenesis of thrombocytopenia and thrombocytopathia in CME. Other mechanisms involved in the development of thrombocytopenia in CME include increased platelet consumption, splenic sequestration and shortened platelet life span during the acute phase, and decreased production in the chronic phase. Recently, circulating immune-complexes were demonstrated in sera of dogs naturally and experimentally infected with *E. canis*, suggesting that some pathological and clinical manifestations in CME are immune-complex mediated.

Clinical signs

E. canis infects all breeds; however, the German Shepherd Dog appears to be more susceptible to clinical CME. Moreover the disease in this breed appears to be more severe than in other breeds, with a higher mortality rate. There is no predilection for age and both genders are equally affected. The disease is manifested by a wide variety of clinical signs. Factors involved include differences in pathogenicity between *E. canis* strains, breed of dog, co-infections with other arthropod-borne pathogens and the immune status of the host.

The clinical signs in the acute phase range from mild and non-specific to severe and life threatening. Common non-specific signs in this phase include depression, lethargy, anorexia, pyrexia, tachypnoea and weight loss. Specific clinical signs include lymphadenomegaly, splenomegaly, petechiation and ecchymoses of the skin and

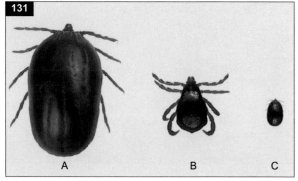

131 An engorged female (A), male (B) and nymph (C) of the brown dog tick *Rhipicephalus sanguineus*.

mucous membranes, and occasional epistaxis (**132, 133**). Less commonly reported clinical signs include vomiting, serous to purulent oculonasal discharge and dyspnoea.

The signs in the chronic severe form of the disease may be similar to those seen in the acute disease, but with greater severity. In addition, pale mucous membranes, emaciation and peripheral oedema, especially of the hind-limbs and scrotum, may also occur. Secondary bacterial and protozoal infections, interstitial pneumonia and renal failure may occur during the chronic severe disease. Some reproductive disorders have also been associated with chronic CME. These include prolonged bleeding during oestrus, infertility, abortion and neonatal death.

Ocular signs have been reported to occur during the acute and chronic phases and involve nearly every structure of the eye. Conjunctivitis, conjunctival or iridal petechiae and ecchymoses, corneal oedema, panuveitis and hyphaema have been reported (**134, 135**). Subretinal haemorrhage and retinal detachment resulting in blindness may occur due to a monoclonal gammopathy and hyperviscosity.

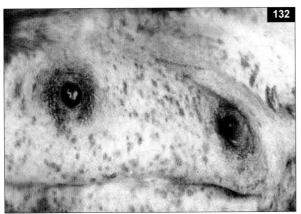
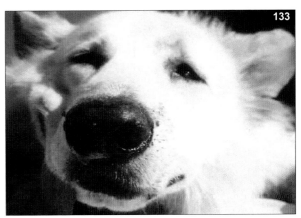

132, 133 Petechiae and ecchymoses (**132**) and epistaxis (**133**) in dogs suffering from CME.

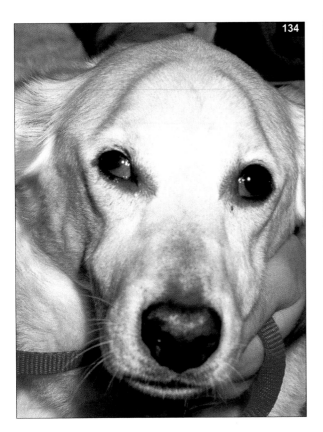
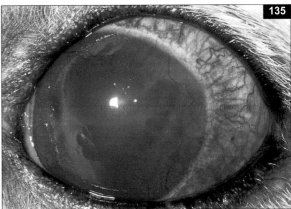

134, 135 A four-year-old Labrador Retriever with secondary glaucoma, episcleral and conjunctival congestion, corneal neovascularization, corneal oedema and iris bombé secondary to *E. canis* infection. (Photos courtesy Dr D Gould) (**135** from *Journal of Small Animal Practice* (2000) **41**, 263–265, with permission)

Neurological signs may occur during both the acute and chronic disease. The signs associated include ataxia, seizures, paresis, hyperasthesia, cranial nerve deficits and vestibular (central or peripheral) signs. Neurological signs may be attributed to meningitis or meningoencephalitis, as evidenced by the extensive lymphoplasmacytic and monocytic infiltration, perivascular cuffing and gliosis. On rare occasions, morulae may be detected in the cerebrospinal fluid of dogs with neurological signs.

A recent small case series suggested that *E. canis* might infect cats. The clinical signs in the three suspected cats included anorexia, lethargy, fever, pale mucous membranes, joint pain, lymphadenomegaly and petechial haemorrhages.

Diagnosis

Diagnosis of CME is based on compatible history, clinical presentation and clinical pathological findings in combination with serology, PCR or *in vitro* culturing of the rickettsial organism. Living in an endemic area or travelling to such an area and/or a history of tick infestation should increase the suspicion of infection with *E. canis*. The importance of early diagnosis lies in the relatively good response to treatment before the dogs enter the chronic phase.

Haematology and blood smear evaluation

Intracytoplasmic *E. canis* morulae may be visualized in monocytes during the acute phase of the disease in about 4% of cases (**129**) and their presence is diagnostic of CME. In order to increase the chance of visualizing morulae, buffy-coat smears should be performed and carefully evaluated (see Chapters 4 and 6).

Thrombocytopenia is the most common and consistent haematological finding in CME. A concurrent increase in the mean platelet volume is usually seen in the acute phase, and megaplatelets appear in the blood smear, reflecting active thrombopoiesis. Mild leucopenia and anaemia may also occur in the acute phase. Absolute monocytosis and the presence of reactive monocytes and large granular lymphocytes are typical findings in acute CME. Mild thrombocytopenia is a common finding in the subclinical phase of the disease, while severe pancytopenia is the hallmark of the severe chronic phase, occurring as a result of a suppressed hypocellular bone marrow.

Serum biochemistry

Hypoalbuminaemia and hyperglobulinaemia are the principal biochemical abnormalities seen in dogs infected with CME. The hyperglobulinaemia is mainly due to hypergammaglobulinaemia. The hypergammaglobulinaemia in CME is usually polyclonal, as determined by serum protein electrophoresis. On rare occasions, monoclonal gammopathy may be noticed and may result in a hyperviscosity syndrome (**136**). Pancytopenic dogs reveal significantly lower concentrations of total protein, total globulin and gammaglobulin compared to non-pancytopenic dogs. Mild transient increases in serum ALT and ALP activities may also be present.

Antiplatelet antibody test as well as Coombs test may be positive in infected dogs. Circulating immune complexes may also be demonstrated; however, anti-nuclear antibodies are not detected in *E. canis* infected dogs.

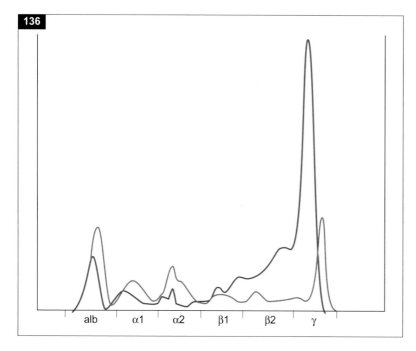

136 Serum protein electrophoresis from the dog shown in **134** and **135**. At the time of presentation (blue) there is a monoclonal gammopathy, the severity of which was reduced after treatment (red). (From *Journal of Small Animal Practice* (2000) **41**, 263–265, with permission)

Specific tests

The IFA test is the most widely used serological assay for the diagnosis of canine ehrlichiosis (137). It is considered the serological 'gold standard' for the detection and titration of *E. canis* antibodies. The presence of *E. canis* antibody titres at a dilution equal to or greater than 1:40 is considered evidence of exposure. Two consecutive tests are recommended, 1–2 weeks apart. A fourfold increase in the antibody titre indicates active infection. In areas that are endemic for other *Ehrlichia* species, serological cross-reactivity may confound the diagnosis. Cross-reactivity between *E. canis* and *E. ewingii*, *E. chaffeensis*, *A. phagocytophilum*, *N. risticii* and *N. helminthoeca* has been documented and should be taken into consideration. There is no serological cross-reaction between *E. canis* and *A. platys* (*Table 32*).

Immunoblot analysis demonstrates that immune sera obtained from infected dogs react with the major antigenic proteins (MAP) of *E. canis* that have a molecular weight of 28–30 kDa. Conventional ELISAs for *E. canis* IgG antibodies have been developed and are useful in detecting *E. canis* antibodies. Recently, an ELISA test using the *E. canis* recombinant MAP2, a 26 kDa protein, as an antigen has been developed and shown to be effective. Several sensitive and specific commercial dot-ELISA tests for *E. canis* antibodies, designed for rapid in-clinic use, have been developed. These include assays that use the whole cultured rickettsia or specific *E. canis* proteins (p 30 and p 30/31) as a source of antigen.

Other methods used in diagnosing *E. canis* infections are culturing the organism on macrophage cell lines (DH82 or J774.A1) (138) and PCR using specific primers for *E. canis*. Both these methods require sophisticated equipment.

Concurrent infections of *E. canis* with other tick-borne pathogens such as *Babesia* species and *Hepatozoon canis* are common. Therefore, it is important microscopically to examine blood smears of infected dogs and to consider multiple serological or PCR screening for co-infecting organisms.

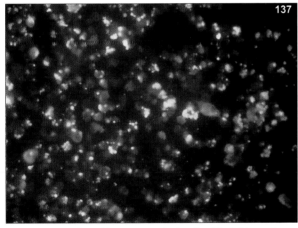

137 IFA assay. A positive test result showing *Ehrlichia canis* morulae detected by overlaying seropositive patient serum and fluorescein-conjugated anti-dog IgG.

138 Multiple *Ehrlichia canis* morulae in the cytoplasm of a tissue culture cell (DH82 macrophage). (Giemsa stain, original magnification ×1,000)

Table 32 Serological cross-reactivity of ehrlichial organisms with *E. canis* antigen.

Ehrlichial agent	Serological IFA cross-reactivity with *E. canis*
E. chaffeensis	+++
E. ewingii	++/+++
VHE/VDE* agent	+++
A. phagocytophilum	–/+
A. platys	–
N. helminthoeca	++
N. risticii	+

– = no cross-reaction; + = weak cross-reaction; ++ = intermediate cross-reaction; +++ = strong cross-reaction; * = Venezuela human *Ehrlichia*/Venezuela dog *Ehrlichia*

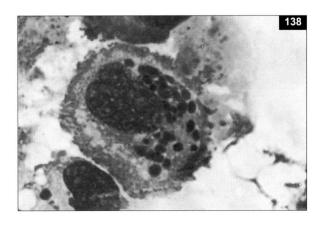

Treatment and control

Doxycycline (10 mg/kg p/o q24h or 5 mg/kg p/o q12h, for a minimum period of 2–3 weeks) is the treatment of choice for acute CME. Seven-day treatment with doxycycline has been shown to be ineffective. Although ten-day treatment has shown success in several studies, in the authors' experience, ten-day treatment may not be sufficient for all acute cases. Most acute cases respond to treatment and show clinical improvement within 24–72 hours. Dogs in the subclinical phase may need prolonged treatment. Treatment of dogs suffering from the chronic severe form of the disease is unrewarding.

Imidocarb dipropionate has previously been used in conjunction with doxycycline in the treatment of CME. Although previous studies have shown the *in vivo* efficacy of imidocarb against *E. canis*, recent *in vivo* and *in vitro* studies using molecular assays have indicated that this drug may not be effective. Nevertheless, the use of imidocarb is indicated when concurrent infections with other protozoa such as *Babesia* species and/or *Hepatozoon canis* are diagnosed. Other drugs with known efficacy against *E. canis* include tetracycline hydrochloride (22 mg/kg q8h), oxytetracycline (25 mg/kg q8h), minocycline (20 mg/kg q12h) and chloramphenicol (50 mg/kg q8h).

After treatment, *E. canis* antibody titres may persist for months and even for years. The persistence of high antibody titres for extended periods may represent an aberrant immune response or treatment failure, but a progressive decrease in the gammaglobulin concentrations is associated with elimination of the organism. *E. canis* antibodies do not provide protection against re-challenge, and seropositive dogs remain susceptible to infection after successful treatment.

To date, no effective anti-*E. canis* vaccine has been developed and tick control remains the most effective preventive measure against infection. In endemic areas, low-dose oxytetracycline treatment (6.6 mg/kg q24h) has been suggested as a prophylactic measure. Recently this method has been used with success by the French army in Senegal, Ivory Coast and Djibouti, where dogs were treated prophylactically with oral oxytetracycline (250 mg/dog p/o q24h). The estimated failure rate of the treatment was found to be 0.9%. This prophylactic method should be reserved for cases where all other prophylactic measures have failed, and should be applied with great caution.

Zoonotic potential/public health significance

In the years 1987–1991 *E. canis* was suspected to infect humans, until a closely related organism named *E. chaffeensis* was identified as the cause of human ehrlichial disease. *E. canis* is not considered a zoonotic agent. However, an *E. canis*-like agent was isolated from a man in Venezuela in 1996, suggesting that the zoonotic potential of *E. canis* has yet to be fully elucidated.

OTHER ERHLICHIA: *EHRLICHIA CHAFFEENSIS*

Background, aetiology and epidemiology

E. chaffeensis, the cause of human monocytic ehrlichiosis (HME), was first isolated from a human patient in 1991. The organism has been convincingly identified from humans, deer, dogs and ticks only in the USA, mainly in the south-central, southeastern and mid-Atlantic states and California. Detection of *E. chaffeensis* DNA by PCR amplification provided evidence for natural canine *E. chaffeensis* infection in southeastern Virginia, Oklahoma and North Carolina.

E. chaffeensis is transmitted by *Amblyomma americanum* (the lone star tick) and, to a lesser extent, by *D. variabilis*. Persistently infected white-tailed deer (*Odocoileus virginianus*) and, possibly, canines serve as reservoirs.

Clinical signs

Pups experimentally infected with *E. chaffeensis* have shown fever and no other signs. Only one report has suggested that *E. chaffeensis* may cause severe clinical signs in dogs, and the clinical significance of natural canine infection has yet to be determined.

Diagnosis

The IFA test is a good screening test for exposure to rickettsiae; however, it cannot differentiate between *E. canis*, *E. chaffeensis* and *E. ewingii* antibodies. It is possible to discriminate between the three species by western immunoblot analysis and by PCR using species-specific primers.

Treatment and control

Tetracyclines, especially doxycycline, are considered the drugs of choice. Control of infection is based solely on optimal application of acaricides or tick removal.

Zoonotic potential/public health significance

E. chaffeensis infects humans and causes HME. Frequent presenting symptoms are fever, malaise, headache, myalgia, chills, diaphoresis, nausea and anorexia. HME may be fatal. The role of dogs as zoonotic reservoirs for infection with *E. chaffeensis* has not been established.

EHRLICHIA EWINGII

Background, aetiology and epidemiology

Although classified in the *E. canis* genogroup, *E. ewingii* infects granulocytes, causing a granulocytic ehrlichiosis in canines. Based on 16S rRNA gene sequence, *E. ewingii* is most closely related to *E. chaffeensis* (98.1%) and *E. canis* (98.0%). *E. ewingii* has not yet been cultured *in vitro*.

Ehrlichiosis caused by *E. ewingii* has been diagnosed in the USA only. It occurs mainly in the spring and early summer. *E. ewingii* has been identified in a large variety of ticks including *R. sanguineus*, *A. americanum*, *D. variabilis*, *Ixodes scapularis* and *I. pacificus*. Of these tick species *A. americanum* is the only proven vector for *E. ewingii*. The role of the other tick species in transmission of the organism warrants further investigation.

Clinical signs
The disease is usually an acute mild disease that can lead to polyarthritis in chronically infected dogs. Lameness, joint swelling, stiff gait and fever are common clinical signs.

Diagnosis
Haematological changes in *E. ewingii* infection are mild and include thrombocytopenia and anaemia. Identification of ehrlichial morulae in neutrophils in peripheral blood or joint effusions is diagnostic of granulocytic ehrlichiosis. However, western immunoblot and PCR using species-specific ehrlichial primers should be used to confirm the ehrlichial species. Species determination is important as *A. phagocytophilum* is also associated with intraneutrophilic morula formation and similar clinical signs in dogs. As *E. ewingii* has not yet been cultured *in vitro*, antigen is not readily available for IFA test development. *E. ewingii* antibodies strongly cross-react with *E. canis* and *E. chaffeensis*, and do not (or weakly) react with *A. phagocytophilum*. Therefore, demonstration of granulocytic ehrlichial morulae and negative serology for *A. phagocytophilum* should increase the suspicion of infection with *E. ewingii*. In such situations, PCR for acute cases would be the preferred diagnostic test. However, in the chronic stage of the disease, western blotting may assist in diagnosing the agent.

Treatment and control
Tetracycline and, especially, doxycycline elicit rapid clinical improvement. As for the other ehrlichioses, prophylaxis is based on tick control.

Zoonotic potential/public health significance
E. ewingii has recently been implicated as the cause of human infections in the USA, particularly in immunocompromised people. The role of the dog as a zoonotic reservoir for *E. ewingii* infection is unknown.

PART 2: GRANULOCYTIC EHRLICHIOSIS: *ANAPLASMA PHAGOCYTOPHILUM* COMB.NOV (*E. PHAGOCYTOPHILA* GENOGROUP) INFECTION

Anneli Bjöersdorff

Background, aetiology and epidemiology
The reclassified species *Anaplasma phagocytophilum* comb.nov comprises the previously separate species of *E. phagocytophila*, *E. equi* and the human granulocytic ehrlichiosis agent (HE agent).

A. phagocytophilum comb.nov (*A. phagocytophilum*) are tick-borne rickettsial microorganisms primarily infecting granulocytes. They cause 'tick-borne fever', an acute febrile disease originally described in the early 1930s in Scottish sheep. During the 1950s and 1960s the microorganisms were reported from England and Finland, respectively, as a cause of 'pasture fever' in cattle. Ehrlichiosis in dogs due to *A. phagocytophilum* was reported from Switzerland, Sweden and North America in the 1980s. Granulocytic ehrlichiosis in cats was first reported from Sweden in the late 1990s and has now also been reported from the UK, Denmark and North America.

A. phagocytophilum are obligate intracellular bacteria infecting cells of bone marrow derivation. They are internalized in phagosomes by the host cell and appear within the cytoplasm as membrane-bound vacuoles (**139**). The bacteria multiply by binary fission and eventually form large inclusion bodies (morulae). In untreated animals the cytoplasmic inclusions can be detected in circulating neutrophils for 1–2 weeks.

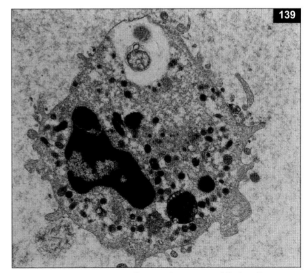

139 Electron micrograph of an equine neutrophil showing *Anaplasma* organisms inside a cytoplasmic vacuole.

Rodents, as well as domestic and wild ruminants (sheep and deer), have been reported as reservoir hosts of *A. phagocytophilum* in Europe. The predominant reservoir host varies depending on the local natural and agricultural landscape. The vector of *A. phagocytophilum* in Europe is the common hard-bodied tick *Ixodes ricinus*. *A. phagocytophilum* spend part of their normal life cycle within the tick and are transmitted trans-stadially. As *I. ricinus* feed on a wide range of vertebrate animals, transmission of the infectious agent may take place to multiple host species. Vector to host transmission is thought to occur within a narrow window of 40–48 hours of feeding.

Pathogenesis

The pathogenesis of granulocytic ehrlichiosis is not clear. Organisms enter the dermis via tick-bite inoculation and are then spread via the blood and/or the lymph. *A. phagocytophilum* is seen in mature granulocytes, mainly in neutrophils but also in eosinophils, of the peripheral blood. However, it is not clear whether the organisms invade mature cells or precursor cells within the myelopoietic system. The adhesion molecule P-selectin that is expressed on the neutrophil surface may act as a receptor for the organism but the bacterial ligand for this receptor is unknown. After endocytosis, the bacteria multiply within cytoplasmic phagosomes. An important virulence factor of *A. phagocytophilum* is the ability to prevent phagosome-lysosome fusion within the cell and thereby evade degradation.

The first cytoplasmic inclusions can be detected in peripheral blood granulocytes of dogs 4–14 days after experimental infection. Immunohistological studies demonstrate the presence of *A. phagocytophilum* in phagocytes in many organs (e.g. spleen, lungs and liver). Localized infection has also been seen in kidney and heart. Infection of endothelial cells by *A. phagocytophilum* has also been reported. Endogenous bacterial pyrogens have not been described in experimental infections. It has been speculated that the pathogenesis of ehrlichiosis is not entirely caused by the organism itself but that injury may be in part host-mediated. Severe pulmonary inflammation, alveolar damage and vasculitis of the extremities in the absence of bacterial organisms suggest an immunopathological course of events, such as cytokine-mediated stimulation of host macrophages and non-specific mononuclear phagocyte activity. The infection may also induce an overactive inflammatory response such as a septic shock-like syndrome, or diffuse alveolar damage leading to respiratory distress syndrome. Phagocytic dysfunction of infected neutrophils may result in a defective host defence and subsequent secondary infections have been reported. Persistent *A. phagocytophilum* infection has been demonstrated in experimentally infected, untreated dogs for up to five-and-a-half months after inoculation.

As *I. ricinus* ticks may harbour and transmit many pathogens, co-infection with two or more pathogens is possible. Both animals and humans can be co-infected with various *Anaplasma*, *Ehrlichia*, *Borrelia*, *Bartonella*, *Rickettsia*, *Babesia* and arboviral species. Infection with any of these organisms causes a wide range of clinical and pathological abnormalities, ranging in severity from asymptomatic infection to death. The risk of acquiring one or more tick-borne infections may be dependent on the prevalence of multi-infected vectors. It has been shown that ticks dually infected with *A. phagocytophilum* and *Borrelia burgdorferi* transmit each pathogen to susceptible hosts as efficiently as ticks infected with only one pathogen. The presence of either agent in the tick does not affect acquisition of the other agent from an infected host. Since *Borrelia burgdorferi* and *A. phagocytophilum* to a large extent share both reservoir hosts and vectors, it is hardly surprising that the geographic areas where granulocytic ehrlichiosis is endemic overlap with areas where borreliosis is prevalent.

The general capacity of one tick-borne infection to predispose to or aggravate another infection is not clear. However, infection with *A. phagocytophilum* has been shown to predispose sheep to disease of increased severity upon exposure to parainfluenza type-3 virus or louping-ill virus. In addition, concurrent *A. phagocytophilum* and *Babesia* infection can result in aggravated disease manifestations in humans.

Clinical signs

The spectrum of clinical manifestations caused by *A. phagocytophilum* is wide but disease most commonly presents as an acute febrile syndrome. The incubation period may vary from 4–14 days depending on the immune status of the infected individual and the bacterial strain involved. Dogs with granulocytic ehrlichiosis usually present with a history of lethargy and anorexia. The clinical examination commonly reveals fever, reluctance to move and, occasionally, splenomegaly (140). More localized presenting signs referable to the musculoskeletal system (lameness), gastrointestinal

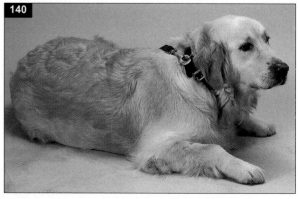

140 A one-year-old, female Golden Retriever with acute granulocytic ehrlichiosis (anaplasmosis). The dog showed pyrexia, weakness and lameness due to polyarthritis.

system (diarrhoea) or central nervous system (seizures or proprioceptive deficits) may be seen. Systemic manifestations may include haemorrhage, shock and multi-organ failure. However, seroepidemiological data suggest that mild and subclinical infections are common.

Laboratory findings

Laboratory investigations of value include white blood cell count, platelet count and hepatic transaminase levels. During and after the period of bacteraemia, the disease is characterized by major haematological changes typified by thrombocytopenia and leucopenia (**141**). The leucopenia is a result of early lymphopenia later accompanied by neutropenia. The leucopenia is followed by transient leucocytosis. Thrombocytopenia is one of the most consistent haematological abnormalities in infected dogs. It may be moderate to severe and persists for a few days before returning to normal. Biochemical abnormalities may include mildly elevated SAP and ALT activities.

141 Serial changes in a range of parameters in a dog experimentally infected with a Swedish *Ehrlichia* (*Anaplasma*) isolate and monitored for a 25-day period. The dramatic haematological changes during the acute stage of infection may be seen. (From *Veterinary Record* (1998) **143**, 412–417, with permission)

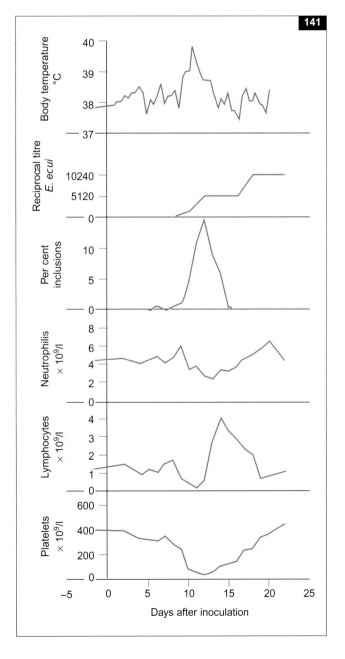

Diagnosis

Granulocytic ehrlichiosis should be considered when a patient presents with an acute febrile illness in a geographic area endemic for the disease, during a season when ticks are host seeking. The Center for Disease Control (Atlanta, USA) case definition adapted for granulocytic ehrlichiosis in dogs and cats is given in *Table 33*.

As intracytoplasmic clusters of the bacteria (morulae) may be visible, a Wright's-stained blood smear should be examined. Morulae typically appear as dark blue, irregularly stained densities in the cytoplasm of neutrophils. The colour of the morulae is usually darker than that of the cell nucleus (**142**). Morulae are often sparse and difficult to detect and a negative blood smear cannot rule out *A. phagocytophilum* infection.

Specific diagnostic tests include anti-*A. phago-cytophilum* IgG and IgM antibody evaluation (IFAs, immunoblot analyses and ELISA) and PCR analyses (**143**). Some research laboratories also offer the service of *in-vitro* culture for *Anaplasma* (**144**). The most widely accepted diagnostic criterion is a fourfold change in titre by IFA (**145**). However, cross-reactivity may occur with other members of the genera *Anaplasma* and *Ehrlichia* (*Table 32*, p. 125).

PCR analysis using *A. phagocytophilum*-specific primers is a very sensitive and specific method for establishing the cause of an infection. PCR is more sensitive than direct microscopy, and *Anaplasma* are detected in the circulation for a longer time period by PCR compared with microscopy. In addition to blood, synovial fluid, cerebrospinal fluid and tissue samples may be analysed by PCR.

Table 33 Case definition of acute canine and feline granulocytic ehrlichiosis.
(Adapted from Centers for Disease Control and Prevention, 2000)

Clinical description
A tick-borne, febrile illness most commonly characterized by acute onset. Clinical laboratory findings may include intracytoplasmic bacterial aggregates (morulae) in leukocytes of a peripheral blood smear, cytopenias (especially thrombocytopenia and leukopenia) and elevated liver enzymes.

Laboratory criteria for diagnosis
- Demonstration of a fourfold or greater change in antibody titre to *A. phagocytophilum* antigen by IFA in acute- and convalescent-phase serum samples, ideally taken greater than or equal to four weeks apart, **or**
- Positive PCR assay and confirmation of *A. phagocytophilum* DNA, **or**
- Identification of morulae in leukocytes in blood, bone marrow or CSF, and a positive IFA titre *to A. phagocytophilum* antigen (based on cut-off titres established by the laboratory performing the assay), **or**
- Culture of *A. phagocytophilum* from a clinical specimen.

Case description
- Probable: a clinically compatible illness with either a single positive IFA titre (based on cut-off titres established by the laboratory performing the test) or the visualization of morulae in leukocytes.
- Confirmed: a clinically compatible illness that is laboratory-confirmed.

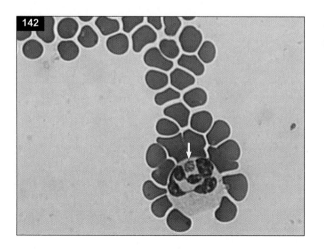

142 *A. phagocytophilum* inclusion (morula) in a neutrophil (arrowed).

143 Comparison of microscopy (a), PCR (b) and serology (c) in an experimental infection of a dog with a Swedish *Ehrlichia* (*Anaplasma*) isolate. The dog was administered prednisolone on days 55 and 153 and was monitored for a 180-day period. It can be seen that persistent infection results in prolonged seropositivity that does not discriminate the cyclical infection demonstrated by PCR. (From *Veterinary Record* (2000) **146**, 186–190, with permission)

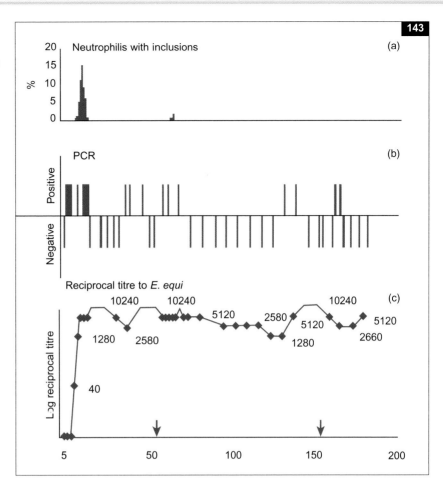

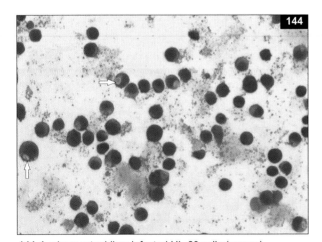

144 *A. phagocytophilum*-infected HL-60 cells (arrows).

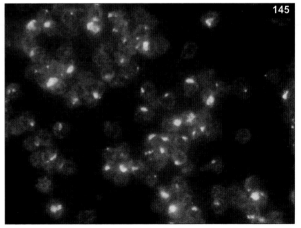

145 IFA test showing positivity for *A. phagocytophilum*. A whole cell *A. phagocytophilum* antigen is often used in diagnostic IFA. The primary antibody–antigen reaction is demonstrated by the use of a secondary fluorescein-labelled antibody. If the serum sample contains antibodies to the antigen, strong fluorescence is seen.

Treatment and control

In vitro, A. phagocytophilum is susceptible to several intracellularly active antibiotics including tetracyclines, rifampicin, rifabutin and trovafloxacin. *A. phagocytophilum* is resistant to gentamicin, erythromycin, azithromycin, clindamycin and trimethoprim-sulphamethoxazole, and to all antibiotics that do not penetrate intracellularly including the β-lactam antibiotics. However, *in-vivo* effects have only been documented for tetracyclines and, to some extent, for rifampicin and chloramphenicol. Doxycycline (5–10 mg/kg q24h for 10 days to 3 weeks) appears to be the most effective regime for treating granulocytic ehrlichiosis in dogs and cats. Severe disease may require treatment for longer periods. In young animals with granulocytic ehrlichiosis, doxycycline is still considered the drug of first choice. The risks of enamel hypoplasia and discoloration are considered low when balanced against the risk of serious infection. The most common side-effects of doxycycline treatment are nausea and vomiting, which are avoided by administering the drug with food. Simultaneous feeding does not affect drug absorption.

Treatment using the anti-protozoal drug imidocarb dipropionate in *E. equi*-seropositive dogs with long-standing clinical signs has been evaluated. The dogs were all non-responsive to previous doxycycline therapy. After follow-up periods ranging from four months to 4.5 years post imidocarb dipropionate treatment, 62% showed a favourable response.

No vaccines for protection or immunoglobulins for postexposure prophylaxis are available. The most reliable, although not the most realistic way, to prevent infections is to avoid tick-infested areas. Careful daily inspection for and removal of ticks is recommended in combination with the application of residual acaricidal products. Spray, spot-on liquid or collar formulations are available with residual efficacy of one month or more depending on the product.

Zoonotic potential/public health significance

The catholic feeding behaviour of the tick vector *I. ricinus* permits transmission of *A. phagocytophilum* to a wide range of vertebrate species including humans. In spite of this fact, less than 50 cases of human infection have so far been reported from Europe. The majority of cases of human granulocytic ehrlichiosis (HGE) have been reported from the USA, where HGE is regarded as a significant emerging tick-borne infection. The most common clinical manifestations of human ehrlichiosis are fever and headache. The clinical disease is often accompanied by non-specific symptoms such as myalgia, stiffness, malaise and arthralgia. Symptoms implicating involvement of other organ systems are also present and include gastrointestinal (nausea, vomiting, diarrhoea), respiratory (non-productive cough) and central nervous system signs (confusion). Skin rashes are uncommonly reported and involvement of concurrent infectious agents has been suggested in these cases. However, it may well be a part of the host inflammatory response to infection. Laboratory data frequently demonstrate thrombocytopenia, leucopenia and elevated levels of hepatic transaminases. Severe complications include prolonged fever, shock, seizures, pneumonitis, acute renal failure, rhabdomyolysis, opportunistic infections, adult respiratory distress syndrome (ARDS) and death. Pre-existing immune dysfunction predisposes to poor prognosis and the risk of serious illness or death increases with advanced age and delayed onset of therapy.

A wide spectrum of symptoms has also been found in European cases, despite seroprevalence data suggesting that the infection is often mild and self-resolving. Fatal infections have not been reported to date in Europe.

PART 3: INFECTIOUS CANINE CYCLIC THROMBOCYTOPENIA: *ANAPLASMA PLATYS* COMB. NOV INFECTION

Susan Shaw

Background, aetiology and epidemiology

Canine cyclic thrombocytopenia, caused by *Anaplasma (E.) platys,* was first described in the USA but has a worldwide distribution. It has been reported from southern Europe, Israel, southeastern and eastern Asia, Venezuela and, most recently, Australia. The aetiological agent is an obligate, intracellular rickettsial organism with tropism for mature platelets. Although originally referred to as *Ehrlichia platys*, based on phenotypic similarities to other organisms of this genus, it has recently been formally classified according to its 16S rRNA gene sequence as a member of the genus *Anaplasma*. Although *A. platys* is predominantly reported from domesticated dogs, the extent of its host spectrum has not been fully determined. Similar organisms have been reported from North American deer and from sheep species in South Africa.

A. platys organisms are round to oval in shape, vary in size from 0.3–1.2 μm in diameter, and are enclosed by a double membrane. The mechanism by which organisms attach and penetrate platelet membranes is unknown. *A. platys* bacteria aggregate and divide within membrane-bound vacuoles within platelet cytoplasm, producing the morulae identified on light microscopy. Further bacteriological characterization is limited, as the organism remains unculturable.

Infection with *A. platys* is presumed to be transmitted by the tick *Rhipicephalus sanguineus*, and its widespread geographic distribution supports this mode of transmission. In particular, *R. sanguineus* is the only tick species that has been identified in isolated areas of central Australia where *A. platys* infection has been reported. In addition, co-infection with *Ehrlichia canis*, which is known to be transmitted by *R. sanguineus*, is reported from several areas of the world. *A. platys* DNA has been identified in *R. sanguineus* ticks collected from dogs in Japan but definitive evidence of natural transmission is still lacking and experimental transmission by *R. sanguineus* has not been successful.

There is limited information available on other epidemiological aspects of *A. platys* infection, although studies would suggest that the prevalence is relatively high in some dog populations. Using IFA testing, seropositivity in two southern states of the USA was widespread; 33% of thrombocytopenic dogs in endemic areas were positive. In addition, 13/28 apparently healthy dogs sampled from one study site in northern Australia were positive for *A. platys* DNA by PCR. Although puppies may be more susceptible to clinical *A. platys* infection in northern Australia, there are no breed, gender, individual predispositions or risk factors for infection reported. However, as mentioned below, concurrent infection with other arthropod-borne infections is a considerable risk factor for the clinical expression of infection. Up to 50% of dogs seropositive for *A. platys* in one USA study were concurrently seropositive for *E. canis*.

Pathogenesis

In dogs the period of time from experimental inoculation of *A. platys* to the appearance of circulating parasitized platelets ranges from 8–15 days. The period of maximum parasitaemia is followed by severe thrombocytopenia, possibly due to direct platelet injury. The number of circulating organisms decreases and recovery in the platelet count occurs within 3–4 days. Repeated episodes of parasitaemia and thrombocytopenia occur at 1–2 week intervals. Although the degree of parasitaemia is much reduced (1% platelets infected) in recurrent episodes, the thrombocytopenia remains severe. Immune-mediated platelet destruction is a more likely mechanism for thrombocytopenia during this phase. Chronic infection is associated with cyclic low-level parasitaemia and mild thrombocytopenia, which may reflect host–*A. platys* adaptation. Antibody titres may persist for four months to five years.

Clinical signs

Infection with *A. platys* is commonly asymptomatic unless the dog undergoes surgery or has a concurrent bleeding disorder such as that produced by co-infection with *E. canis*. However, there are reports from Greece and Israel of more severe disease associated with infection. Clinical signs include cyclical fever (in the early phases of infection), lymphadenomegaly and bleeding disorders. *A. platys* infection has been associated with cyclical epistaxis and bleeding from venipuncture sites in adult dogs, and severe thrombocytopenia with anaemia and increased mortality rate in puppies seen in northern Australian dogs. Bilateral uveitis has been reported in one dog with *A. platys* infection.

The spectrum of clinical signs is suggestive of geographical strain variation and minor sequence differences have been detected in *A. platys* samples from the USA and Australia.

It is widely accepted that clinical signs associated with *A. platys* infection may be precipitated through co-infection with other arthropod-borne diseases such as babesiosis and ehrlichiosis.

Laboratory findings

Thrombocytopenia is the major haematological finding, although leucopenia has also been reported in rare cases. Cyclical thrombocytopenic episodes of 3–4 days duration, followed by asymptomatic periods of 7–21 days, are characteristic of *A. platys* infection. A moderate non-regenerative anaemia is associated with infectious canine thrombocytopenia, probably as a result of inflammation. However, in the uncommon cases that experience severe bleeding, a regenerative anaemia may be expected. Moderate hypergammaglobulinaemia, occasional hypo-albuminaemia and hypocalcaemia have also been reported.

Diagnosis

The microscopic identification of morulae in platelets, with morphology characteristic of *A. platys* in stained blood smears, is diagnostic for infection. However, the sensitivity of this technique is greatly limited by the low levels of parasitaemia seen during severe thrombo-cytopenic episodes and in chronic infections. Attempts to culture *A. platys* have been uniformly unsuccessful.

Serology has been the major technique used for *A. platys* diagnosis. IFA testing for *A. platys* has been developed but its availability is currently severely limited by lack of antigen substrate. Cross-reactions with *E. canis* reportedly do not occur but cross-reactivity with *A. phagocytophilum* has not been investigated.

Several methods of species-specific PCR testing are available and, considering the limitations of serology and microscopy in the diagnosis of this infection, they are sensitive and specific adjuncts to diagnosis.

Treatment and control

Although specific recommendations for treatment have not been determined, *A. platys* infection should be treated with tetracyclines using protocols discussed for other members of the genera *Ehrlichia* and *Anaplasma*. Prevention is dependent on vector control using effective acaricides with long duration.

Zoonotic potential/public health significance

Currently, there are no recognized public health implications associated with canine *A. platys* infection.

Rickettsial infections
Craig Greene

TICK-TRANSMITTED RICKETTSIAL INFECTIONS

Introduction

Serologically and pathogenically distinct members of the genus *Rickettsia* exist throughout the world and cause febrile exanthems in people. In the western hemisphere, *Rickettsia rickettsii*, the most important and most pathogenic organism, causes Rocky Mountain spotted fever (RMSF). This disease is important as a potentially fatal illness in people, and dogs are known to be similarly affected. Naturally occurring disease has not been reported in cats. Other closely related non-pathogenic members of the spotted fever group (SFG) in North America are *R. montana*, *R. rhipicephali*, *R. bellii* and *R. canada*. These are thought to produce subclinical infections; however, *R. canada* may have some virulence. Two ticks, *Dermacentor andersoni* and *D. variabilis*, are primarily responsible for transmission of *R. rickettsii* in North America. *Rhipicephalus sanguineus* and *Amblyomma cajennense* are involved in transmission of RMSF in Mexico and South America.

In other parts of the world, similar SFG rickettsial and tick reservoir cycles exist. *R. conorii*, which causes boutonneuse or Mediterranean spotted fever, is an analogous organism to *R. rickettsii*, predominating in Europe, Asia and Africa. It is primarily transmitted by dog ticks of the genus *Rhipicephalus*, and dogs and rodents are the chief hosts. Dogs appear to have subclinical infection but they may facilitate transport of ticks and serve as reservoir hosts for infection of humans. Queensland tick typhus (*R. australis*), Flinder's Island spotted fever (*R. honei*), African tick bite fever (*R. africae*), Astrakhan fever (Astrakhan fever rickettsia), Japanese spotted fever (*R. japonica*), North Asian tick typhus (*R. sibirica*) and unnamed European rickettsioses (*R. helvetica*, *R. mongolotimonae*, *R. slovaca*), are analogous diseases of humans caused by other SFG rickettsiae and transmitted by arthropods in geographically distinct regions. The clinical significance in, or reservoir status of, dogs or cats for these infections in the eastern hemisphere has not been determined.

Rocky Mountain spotted fever

In this section, RMSF, as it occurs in the Americas, is emphasized as the model disease for tick-transmitted SFG rickettsiosis because it is the only infection caused by tick-borne rickettsiae documented to cause clinical illness in dogs or cats.

Ticks become infected with *R. rickettsii* by feeding on small rodents that have sufficient rickettsaemia to allow transmission. Immature ticks become infected and infection is transmitted trans-stadially and transovarially to later tick stages, which feed on larger mammals. Therefore, the disease becomes established in a given geographic region. Despite the presence of adequate hosts and ticks, *R. rickettsii*-infected ticks are limited to a small proportion of ticks in the overall population within an area. This is caused by deleterious effects that the organism has on tick metabolism and antagonism or immunity from co-infecting non-pathogenic rickettsiae. In addition to the low prevalence of infection, *R. rickettsii* in infected ticks are not immediately infectious but reactivate their virulence following tick attachment and uptake of a blood meal at the beginning of the season. Generally, attachment periods of 5–20 hours are required for successful transmission.

Pathogenesis

Once *R. rickettsii* are inoculated into the body, they enter the bloodstream and infect endothelial cells. A widespread vasculitis occurs, as the organisms cause endothelial necrosis and spread to enter new cells. Vascular injury leads to activation of the coagulation and fibrinolytic pathways. Platelet consumption and destruction can be caused by coagulatory and immune-mediated mechanisms, respectively. In serious or long-standing untreated cases, organ systems with endarterial circulation (e.g. the skin, brain, heart and kidneys) may develop multiple foci of necrosis. Severe organ failure occurs less commonly in dogs than in people. Vascular injury leads to leakage of intravascular fluids into extracellular fluid spaces and resultant oedema formation. Fluid accumulation in tissues such as the CNS can cause significant brain oedema, resulting in a progressive mental and cardiorespiratory depression.

Clinical signs

Most dogs develop illness during the warmer months of the year; however, this seasonality is less noticeable at lower latitudes. Fever is one of the most consistent signs of illness. It may develop within several days after tick exposure and is associated with lethargy, mental dullness and inappetence (**146**). Animals develop a stiff gait and show arthralgia and myalgia, as demonstrated by difficulty in rising and eventual reluctance to walk. Lymphadenomegaly of all peripheral lymph nodes is apparent (**147**). Hyperaemia of mucosal surfaces and subcutaneous oedema develop (**148, 149**) and in severely affected animals, dermal necrosis ensues (**150**).

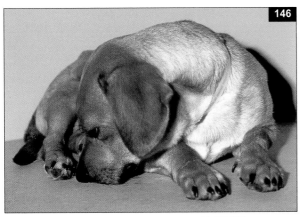

146 Mentally depressed Dachshund dog with RMSF. (Photo courtesy CE Greene)

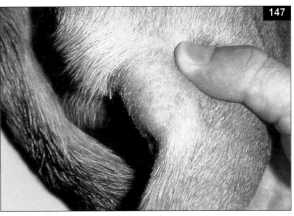

147 Enlarged popliteal lymph node of a Dachshund dog with systemic manifestations of RMSF. (Photo courtesy CE Greene)

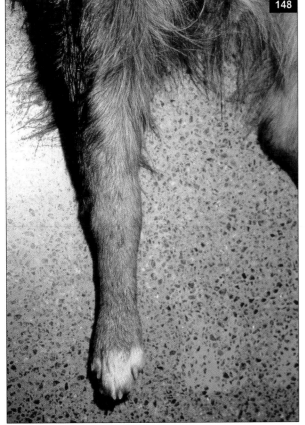

148 Subcutaneous oedema of the limb of a mixed breed dog with RMSF. (Photo courtesy CE Greene)

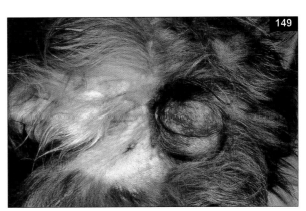

149 Scrotal oedema of the dog in **148**. (Photo courtesy CE Greene)

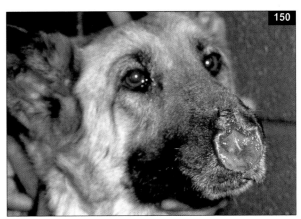

150 Necrosis of the planum nasale in a German Shepherd Dog with RMSF. (Photo courtesy CE Greene)

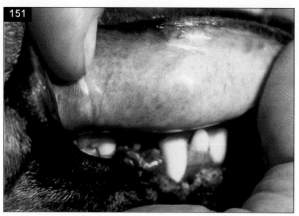

151 Fine petechiae on the lip mucosa of a dog with RMSF. (Photo courtesy CE Greene)

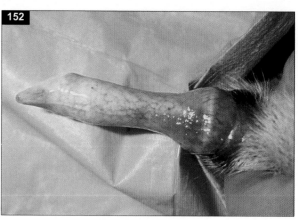

152 Fine petechiae on the penile mucosa of a dog with RMSF. (Photo courtesy CE Greene)

In contrast to the disease in people, dogs infrequently develop petechial haemorrhages, and when they do the distribution is generally on the mucous membranes (**151, 152**). Haemorrhages are also more consistently found in the ocular fundus. Overt haemorrhage is rarely found in the most severely affected animals. Neurological complications often result in animals that suffer a delay in diagnosis and treatment. These are caused by meningitis and can include hyperaesthesia, seizures, vestibular dysfunction and a variety of manifestations depending on the lesion localization. Recovery is rapid and complete in those animals receiving treatment early, before the onset of organ damage or neurological complications. Once the neurological signs have developed, recovery is delayed, or deficits may be permanent.

Diagnosis

Clinical laboratory findings are non-specific for a generalized acute phase inflammatory reaction. Leucopenia in the acute stages is followed by a moderate leucocytosis and stress leucogram. A left shift and toxic granulation of neutrophils may be observed in animals with the most severe tissue necrosis. Thrombocytopenia is one of the most consistent laboratory findings. Coagulation times are usually within normal limits unless dogs develop overt DIC. Serum biochemical abnormalities include hypoalbuminaemia, elevated serum alkaline phosphatase activity and variable hyponatraemia and hyperbilirubinaemia. Analysis of CSF may reveal a mild increase in protein and a neutrophil pleocytosis. Cell counts are increased in joint fluid, with a predominance of neutrophils. Results of tests for autoimmunity are usually negative, with the exception of platelet autoantibody. Electrocardiographic testing may show conduction disturbances related to myocarditis. Thoracic radiography may show a diffuse increase in pulmonary interstitial density.

The microimmunofluorescence (Micro-IF) test is used by most laboratories to determine specific IgG and IgM serum antibodies. When IgM levels are not increased in the initial sample, the most definitive results are obtained by measuring convalescent IgG in sera, collected after a 2–3 week interval. Seronegative results on the first sample do not eliminate the possibility of infection, and a subsequent serum sample should be taken under these conditions. Although inter-laboratory variation exists in measured antibody titres, high IgG levels (e.g. a titre of ≥1024) generally indicate exposure within the last year and may be presumed to mean recent infection if clinical signs are compatible.

Direct immunostaining of tissues has been used for clinical or postmortem diagnosis of RMSF. Full thickness skin biopsies have been submitted to detect the presence of the rickettsiae in dermal blood vessels. This method allows for rapid confirmation of infection; however, it is not widely available and must be performed prior to the administration of antimicrobial therapy. Molecular detection methods (e.g. PCR) have been used to identify rickettsiae in blood or tissue specimens, and nucleic acid may be detected for a period of time after antimicrobial therapy has been instituted. Rickettsial isolation involves risk and can only be done in high bio-containment facilities. At necropsy, pathological lesions include petechial and ecchymotic hemorrhages throughout all body tissues, lymphadenomegaly and splenomegaly. Microscopically, widespread necrotizing vasculitis occurs in many organs.

Treatment and control

Untreated RMSF is a highly fatal disease. Because of the delay in obtaining antibody titres, treatment should be instituted whenever the disease is suspected. Tetracyclines are the antibiotics of choice and treatment should be for at least one week (*Table 34*). Tetracycline is as effective as the more lipid soluble doxycycline, because intracellular penetration is not essential to eliminate the organism. Chloramphenicol and fluoroquinolones have equivalent efficacy, while azithromycin is less effective. Early therapy may delay or suppress the rise in antibody titre of

Table 34 Drug therapy for treatment of spotted fever group rickettsial infections.

Drug	Dose (mg/kg)	Route	Frequency (hours)	Duration (weeks)
Tetracycline	22	P/o	8	1
Doxycycline	5	P/o	12	1
Chloramphenicol	15–30	P/o, s/c, i/v	8	1
Enrofloxacin	3	P/o, s/c	12	1

(Modified from Greene CE, Breitschwerdt EB (1998) Rocky Mountain Spotted Fever. In *Infectious Diseases of the Dog and Cat.* (ed CE Greene) WB Saunders, Philadelphia, with permission)

convalescent samples. Fluid therapy must be restricted because of the danger of causing more oedema in the CNS. Antibiotics are only effective if they are instituted prior to the onset of tissue necrosis or organ failure. The response to treatment, as noted by a reduction in body temperature and improvement in clinical illness, is apparent within 24–48 hours if the diagnosis is correct. Supportive care is needed in dogs with hypotension, coagulopathy or evidence of organ dysfunction.

Recovery from infection is associated with protective immunity against infection with the same rickettsial species. Vaccines are not available commercially, although experimental vaccines have been shown to be protective against severe or prolonged infection. Vaccines containing outer membrane proteins have produced protection against challenge infection in experimental animals.

Prevention is best achieved by strict control of tick vectors and periodic treatment with insecticides. Newer means of tick control for dogs include the use of systemic or topically applied acaricides.

Zoonotic potential/public health significance

RMSF is an important zoonotic disease because of its high prevalence and potentially fatal outcome if diagnosis is delayed or missed. Despite the availability of effective treatment, annual mortality rates approach 5%. Infection rate and seasonality in dogs parallels that in people; however, this is caused by an exposure to the same ticks in the environment. Dogs may be infested with engorged ticks that infect people as they remove them or allow tick excreta or haemolymph to enter abraded skin or mucous membranes. Clinical signs in people are very similar to those in dogs. Early signs in people may be vague and misdiagnosis can occur until a rash develops later in the course of the disease. Most of the fatalities are due to lack of early suspicion and treatment. Care should always be taken in removing attached ticks, and forceps or protective gloves should be used. People should apply tick repellents when spending time in tick-infested areas.

FLEA-TRANSMITTED RICKETTSIAL INFECTIONS

Two causes of flea-transmitted human typhus are now recognized: *Rickettsia typhi*, which is transmitted by rodent fleas and has a worldwide distribution; and the recently reported *R. felis*, which has been identified in cats, dogs and in cat fleas (*Ctenocephalides felis*) in the Americas and Europe to date. In endemic areas of the USA, peri-urban opossums are major reservoir hosts for *R. felis* but the reservoir potential of cats and dogs has not been determined. In North America, *R. typhi* infections have been found in fleas and people in the same geographic areas where *R. felis* exists, although co-infection is not common.

Experimental infection of cats with *R. felis* has been demonstrated, as has seropositivity to *R. typhi*. Cats infected with *R. felis* by repeat exposure to feeding fleas develop a subclinical illness with an incubation period of 2–4 months. However, the pathogenic potential of natural infection with either rickettsial species in dogs and cats is unknown. What is known is that cats and dogs will transport *Ct. felis* into domestic surroundings and, as transovarial and trans-stadial transmission of *R. felis* has shown, a domestic focus of infection for humans could be established.

13 Other arthropod-borne infections of dogs and cats

Susan Shaw

INTRODUCTION

Major arthropod-borne infectious diseases with wide geographical distributions and serious clinical outcomes for dogs and cats have been the subject of preceding chapters of this book. This chapter deals with infections that are associated with:

- Low or sporadic prevalence of disease but where exposure, subclinical infection and zoonotic potential may be high.
- Focal geographical distribution but where there may be high morbidity, mortality and/or zoonotic potential.

YERSINIOSIS (PLAGUE)

Background, aetiology and epidemiology

Plague is caused by the non-spore-forming bacterium *Yersinia pestis*. Localized foci of disease occur in temperate, semi-arid areas throughout the world and infection is maintained in reservoir rodent populations via transmission by rodent fleas (such as *Xenopsylla* species). Epizootic outbreaks of disease occur when *Y. pestis* infection spills over into more highly susceptible small mammal populations. With semi-urban development now extending into endemic areas of plague, there is increasing risk of domestic dogs and, more particularly, cats being infected by bites from rodent fleas acquired during hunting and ingestion of infected small mammals. The cat flea *Ctenocephalides felis* is a relatively ineffective vector for plague transmission.

Pathogenesis

Following an infected flea bite, organisms are phagocytosed by macrophages, which transfer infection to local and regional lymph nodes. The production of a capsular envelope ensures the intracellular survival of *Yersinia*. Lymphadenitis develops and this is followed by dissemination of infection and bacteraemia within 2–6 days. In contrast, after ingestion or inhalation of organisms and entry through a mucous membrane, dissemination and the onset of bacteraemia is more rapid (1–3 days).

Clinical signs

Dogs with plague develop mild febrile illness, with lymphadenomegaly. However, humans and domesticated and wild cats are more susceptible to clinical yersiniosis than dogs. In experimentally infected cats, most develop mild to moderately severe clinical disease, with subsequent recovery, although some develop an acute fulminating and fatal syndrome. Two main clinical syndromes are recognized in naturally infected cats. Bubonic plague is associated with fever, dehydration, weight loss and lymphadenopathy, with abscessation and draining tracts affecting the cervical, retropharyngeal and submandibular lymph nodes. Recovery may occur following this stage or there is haematogenous spread with progression to the often fatal, septicaemic syndrome. Multiple organ involvement, endotoxic shock, oedema and disseminated intravascular coagulation (DIC) with marked leucocytosis are characteristic. In cats, pneumonic involvement during this stage is common and dissemination by aerosol may occur to in-contact humans. Primary pneumonic plague in cats is rare. Less commonly reported clinical signs are vomiting, diarrhoea, tonsillar and lingual lymph node enlargement and necrotic stomatitis.

Diagnosis

Notification of state veterinary or health services may be required in some countries when a case of plague is suspected. Confirmation of diagnosis is made by cytological or histopathological demonstration of bacteria in affected tonsillar tissue or lymph node aspirates, with appropriate Gram and Giemsa staining characteristics. This is followed by culture. Stringent biosafety procedures should be followed in collection and transport of specimens and culture requires a specialist containment laboratory. Serological testing by IFA and demonstration of a rising serum antibody titre provide diagnostic support. PCR is also available in *Yersinia* reference laboratories in various areas of the world.

Treatment and control

The decision to treat animals with plague should always take into consideration the zoonotic risk. In particular, the potential for aerosol spread from pulmonary lesions in infected cats should be evaluated by thoracic radiology. Appropriate protective clothing and gloves should be worn and all contaminated material or surfaces should be disinfected. *Y. pestis* is sensitive to routine disinfectants and a variety of antibiotics, including aminoglycosides, doxycycline, chloramphenicol and fluoroquinolones. Therapy should be continued for a minimum of 21 days (*Table 35*). Doxycycline is most commonly used in the bubonic syndrome and can be used for prophylaxis in exposed, subclinical cats.

Flea control in all in-contact cats and dogs is essential. Safe, effective, residual insecticides combined with insect development inhibitors are available. If used regularly, they will provide excellent vector control. Minimizing access of dogs and cats to infected mammal carcasses is also important. An effective and safe vaccination is not presently available for dogs and cats.

Zoonotic potential/public health significance

Bacteraemic cats are a source for human infection either directly through aerosol spread, bites or scratches or indirectly by transporting infected fleas into the domestic environment. Infection, if recognized early, can be treated effectively with antibiotics but untreated cases may be fatal. Vaccines have been developed but are not commercially available.

TULARAEMIA

Background, aetiology and epidemiology

The aetiological agent of tularaemia in mammals and birds is the tick-transmitted bacterium *Francisella tularensis*. These organisms are distributed throughout the temperate and sub-Arctic areas of the northern hemisphere and there is geographic variation in strain, the species of tick vector and the reservoir hosts involved. Two biovars are recognized and cats are susceptible to both. *F. tularensis tularensis* is distributed throughout North America and is associated with a tick–rabbit cycle. *F. tularensis palearctica* has a broad distribution throughout the northern hemisphere and has a more complex epidemiology involving a hare/rabbit reservoir–tick/mosquito cycle. Tick vectors include species of *Dermacentor*, *Amblyomma*, *Ixodes* and *Haemaphysalis*. Cats may also be infected by ingesting infected rodent or lagomorph prey.

Pathogenesis, clinical signs and diagnosis

Cats appear more susceptible to naturally occurring clinical tularaemia than dogs, and younger cats appear more predisposed. Clinical signs include fever, marked lethargy, anorexia, regional or generalized lymphadenopathy with abscessation, splenomegaly and/or hepatomegaly with abscessation, oral ulceration, leucopenia, icterus and in some cases death. Presumptive diagnosis may be made serologically but confirmation requires culture of infected tissue or body fluids using rigorous biosafety procedures to prevent human infection.

Treatment and control

Therapeutic regimes for feline tularaemia have not been thoroughly investigated and are adapted from human medicine. Aminoglycoside, tetracycline, chloramphenicol and fluoroquinolone antibiotics have been advocated, and these should be administered for a 2–4-week period (*Table 35*).

Zoonotic potential/public health significance

Humans may contract tularaemia by several routes including bites from arthropods, particularly ixodid ticks. In addition, infected domestic cats may transmit tularaemia to humans by bites and scratches, although this is rare. In humans, cutaneous inoculation results in ulceroglandular tularaemia. An initial period of fever, headache, chills, cough and myalgia is followed by a short period (1–3 days) of clinical remission. Ulceration and necrotizing lymphadenitis develop in the second clinical phase. Tularaemia is antibiotic sensitive but ulceroglandular tularaemia may be fatal in up to 5% of cases.

Table 35 Drugs recommended for treatment of bacterial arthropod-borne infectious diseases.

Drug	Infection	Dose rate (mg/kg)	Dose frequency (hours)	Route
Doxycycline	Yersiniosis	5–10	12, decrease to 24	P/o
Oxytetracycline	Tularaemia	10–25	8	P/o, i/v
Erythromycin	Coxiellosis	10–22	12	P/o, i/v
Azithromycin**	Coxiellosis	7–15	8–12	P/o
Chloramphenicol	Yersiniosis, tularaemia	25–50	12–24	I/v, i/m, s/c, p/o
Fluoroquinolones* (e.g. enrofloxacin)	Coxiaellosis, yersiniosis, tularaemia	5–10	24	I/v, i/m, s/c, p/o
Aminoglycosides (e.g. gentamycin)	Yersiniosis, tularaemia	2–4	24	I/m
Rifampicin* **	Coxiellosis	5–10	24	P/o
Trimethoprim/sulphonamide/pyrimethamine	Coxiellosis	15–60	24	P/o

* = used in combination with other antibiotics; ** = not licensed for cats

COXIELLOSIS

Background, aetiology, epidemiology and zoonotic significance

Coxiella burnetii is an extracellular, arthropod-transmitted, spore-forming bacterium, which in cats and dogs produces subclinical infection but in humans causes Q fever, a disease associated with fever, arthralgia, myalgia, hepatitis and respiratory disease. A wide range of wild and domesticated animals are considered reservoir hosts for human infection. In wildlife reservoir cycles, *C. burnetii* is commonly transmitted by arthropod vectors, including ticks. In addition, the sporulated form of *C. burnetii* is highly resistant to environmental extremes and can be spread between hosts by ingestion or aerosol dissemination of infected fluids such as milk, urine and vaginal/uterine secretions, or by ingestion of infected tissues such as placental material. Infected cats are considered important reservoirs for human coxiellosis. *C. burnetii* appears to be frequently carried in the vagina of healthy cats in endemic areas and contact with infected parturient cats is a risk factor for human infection.

Seropositivity to *C. burnetii* ranges between 16% and 20% in populations of stray and companion cats in the USA, Canada and Japan, while lower seroprevalences are reported from Africa. Cross-reactivity between *C. burnetii* and *Bartonella henselae* has been reported in human studies and although this has not been investigated in cats, it may inflate seroprevalence figures for *Coxiella*.

Diagnosis

Diagnosis of active infection with *Coxiella* is made by demonstration of a rising antibody titre, PCR or immunohistochemical techniques.

Treatment and control

Treatment of cats may be required in households where there is increased risk of human infection. *Coxiella* infections are variably susceptible to single agent therapy with macrolides (erythromycin, azithromycin), potentiated sulphonamides and fluoroquinolones for 2–4 weeks duration (*Table 35*, p. 139). Combination therapy of doxycycline and fluoroquinolones with rifampicin may be more effective. Routine control of infection beyond routine hygiene recommended for handling of at-risk animals is not appropriate due to the sporadic nature of human infection.

ARTHROPOD-BORNE VIRAL ENCEPHALITIDES

Background and aetiology

Dogs and cats are susceptible to infection with arthropod-borne RNA viruses of several families. The viruses concerned are naturally maintained in sylvatic cycles involving wild mammalian or bird reservoir hosts, although in some cases domesticated herbivores may become part of the reservoir where habitats overlap. Companion animals and humans become exposed accidentally when they are bitten by infected flies or ticks in high-risk habitats. Although only a small percentage of susceptible dogs and cats develop overt neurological disease, a number of the arthropod-borne viruses cause serious disease in humans.

Flaviviruses have a worldwide distribution and some of these viruses cause diseases of both medical and veterinary importance (e.g. West Nile fever, tick-borne encephalitis (TBE), louping ill and Japanese B encephalitis). Viruses in this group are more likely to be associated with clinical disease in dogs but have not been reported to cause clinical signs in cats. Togaviruses cause equine encephalitis in the western hemisphere and although dogs and occasionally cats are susceptible to subclinical infection, naturally occurring clinical disease has not been reported. Natural infections, albeit through non-arthropod borne routes, with viruses of the families Bunyaviridae (Rift Valley fever) and Orbiviridae (African horse sickness, bluetongue) have also been reported in dogs.

TBE and louping ill

TBE and louping ill viruses are two closely related tick-transmitted flaviviruses that occasionally cause neurological disease in European dogs. The main vector for both is *Ixodes ricinus*, although *I. persculatus* is a vector for TBE in Russia and some Baltic regions. TBE is endemic in areas of central, eastern and northern Europe where climatic and geographical factors are favourable. Reservoir hosts for infection include several species of wild rodents (*Clethrionymys* and *Apodemys* species). TBE virus is transmitted trans-stadially and transovarially and transmission also occurs between *I. ricinus* ticks by co-feeding on *Apodemus* mice in the absence of systemic viraemia. Seropositivity is widespread in companion dogs in endemic areas, although illness is not commonly reported. In addition, experimental infection of dogs with TBE fails reliably to reproduce clinical disease.

Louping ill virus is pathogenic for domesticated herbivores, particularly sheep, and is maintained in a sheep–*I. ricinus* cycle, although wild ground–nesting birds such as red grouse are also involved. Both trans-stadial transmission and transmission by co-feeding ticks on non-viraemic hosts occur. Wolves, dogs and foxes are susceptible to infection but as with TBE, disease is rarely reported. Naturally occurring disease has not been reported in cats with either virus.

Both viruses cause acute neurological disease with a seasonal (spring/summer) occurrence. In areas endemic for louping ill, working sheep dogs and gun dogs are more likely to be exposed and thus develop illness.

Pathogenesis and clinical signs

Both virsues have tropism for the central nervous system after a short period of viraemia. In most cases, infection is eliminated by an active immune response and animals in endemic areas may have detectable antibody titres for life.

The incubation period is short (7–14 days or less). Clinical signs of TBE are referable to multifocal neurological involvement and include fever, gait abnormalities, seizures, paresis and peripheral neuropathies, particularly involving the cranial nerves. Initially, dogs with louping ill have CNS signs of more localized cerebellar dysfunction, with ataxia and tremor. Signs are rapidly progressive, with the development of recumbency, tetraplegia, opisthotonus and death in some cases. Recovery can occur but it is slow and may be associated with residual locomotor and cerebral abnormalities. In a Swedish study, only 8% of seropositive dogs developed clinical signs and of these, most recovered from the initial disease over 2–3 months.

Diagnosis

Clinical signs are not pathognomonic for either viral infection. Clinical pathological parameters and CSF analysis are compatible with non-suppurative meningo-encephalitis. Antemortem diagnosis is most commonly made by demonstrating rising serum antibody titres. Serological testing is only available from specialist laboratories. A single positive test on serum is difficult to associate with disease due to the high exposure rates in endemic areas. However, high titres in CSF compared to serum are supportive for TBE. Histopathological examination of brain tissue reveals neuronal necrosis and perivascular lymphoid cuffing that is particularly prominent in the spinal cord. Viral isolation or immunohistochemistry on brain tissue provides postmortem diagnostic confirmation.

Treatment and management

Supportive and symptomatic therapy during the acute phase of illness is particularly important for recovery of infected animals. No specific anti-viral chemotherapy has been recommended. Aggressive control of tick infestation provides the most effective prevention. In addition, control of louping ill in sheep will decrease the risk for working dogs.

Zoonotic potential/public health significance

Humans are accidentally infected with TBE virus through exposure to infected tick bites in a similar manner to companion dogs, although humans are more susceptible to developing clinical signs. About 10–30% of infected humans, particularly children, develop central nervous system disease. Clinical progression is usually biphasic, with a viraemic phase (malaise, fever, lethargy) followed by a period of clinical remission. Clinical signs are referable to non-suppurative meningitis, meningo-encephalitis or polyradiculoneuritis. Although recovery occurs in most cases, serious neurological or neuropsychiatric sequelae may persist for prolonged periods. Recovery is accompanied by lifelong immunity. Companion dogs are considered a sentinel for human TBE virus infection.

Occasional clinical signs occur in humans infected with louping ill virus. The clinical signs are similar to those seen in TBE, although milder.

Both louping ill and TBE may also have alternative methods of transmission. Outbreaks of louping ill in abattoir workers are reported and TBE can be transmitted through ingestion of infected milk.

West Nile virus encephalitis

West Nile fever is caused by a mosquito-transmitted flavivirus that has been recognized in Europe and Africa for several decades but has recently emerged in North America. It causes neurological disease in humans, horses and certain species of birds, and is primarily maintained in wild bird reservoirs. The role of dogs in the epidemiology of West Nile virus (WNV) is thought to be minor. Wild and domesticated canids are susceptible to natural infection, as shown by seropositivity, but clinical disease is difficult to reproduce experimentally. However, neurological disease associated with WNV has recently been reported in susceptible dogs and a wolf in the USA. Clinical signs included fever, lethargy, ataxia and multifocal central nervous system signs. Histopathological findings were compatible with viral encephalitis and diagnosis was confirmed by immunohistochemistry and *in situ* PCR.

TRYPANOSOMIASIS

Aetiology

Trypanosomiasis is caused by a flagellated arthropod-borne protozoan parasite of the genus *Trypanosoma*. Trypanosomes are maintained in a wide range of domestic and wild animal hosts in south and central America, Africa and Asia. *T. cruzi* has been reported to cause disease in dogs in both North and South America. Although cats are susceptible to infection, there are no reports of disease in this species. *T. cruzi* is transmitted primarily by the cutaneous inoculation of faeces from infected haematophagous *Triatoma* bugs, but infection may also be transmitted by ingestion of infected bugs or infected prey. The protozoan parasites are spread haematogenously and then enter an intracellular phase in macrophages and myocytes, where rapid intracellular multiplication takes place.

Clinical signs

In susceptible dogs, clinical signs develop after 14–17 days. Generalized lymphadenopathy is followed by acute myocarditis, particularly in puppies. Chronic disease is associated with right- and then left-sided congestive heart failure, dysrhythmias, ascites, pleural effusion and pulmonary oedema.

Diagnosis

Diagnosis in the acute stage is made by microscopic identification of the parasites in Wright's- or Giemsa-stained blood smears, particularly those made from the buffy coat/plasma interface in centrifuged samples. However, concentration techniques may be necessary in chronic infections with low level parasitaemia. Organisms may also be identified in lymph node aspirates or from fluid cytologies. Organisms are difficult to identify in the chronic stages of the disease. Isolation using culture is difficult and may require cell culture systems. Several serological tests are available at specialist laboratories but there is cross-reactivity with *Leishmania* species.

Treatment

Nifurtimox has been used for treating acute canine trypanosomiasis and is one of the drugs of choice for humans. The prognosis is guarded as dogs surviving the acute phase usually succumb to congestive heart failure. Supportive therapy is recommended but progression usually leads to death.

Zoonotic potential/public health significance

Human trypanosomiasis due to *T. cruzi* (Chagas' disease) is widespread in central and southern America. It is difficult to treat and causes severe disease. Infected dogs provide a peri-domestic reservoir of infection for the vector and, thus, human infection. Both veterinarians and staff should be aware of the potential risk of transmission by blood from infected dogs.

Appendix

Potential vectors of *Dirofilaria immitis*. (Modified and updated from Ludlam *et al.* [1970] Potential vectors of *Dirofilaria immitis*. *Journal of the American Veterinary Medical Association*, 157: 1354–1359).

Species	Geographic area where larval development in the mosquito has been reported	Species	Geographic area where larval development in the mosquito has been reported
Aedes aegypti	Brazil, Nigeria, USA, Japan	*Anopheles maculopennis*	Europe
Aedes albopictus	Taiwan, Brazil, Italy, Japan	*Anopheles minimus flavirostris*	Philippines
Aedes atropalpus	USA		
Aedes canadensis	USA	*Anopheles plumbeus*	Europe
Aedes caspius	Italy, Spain (**)	*Anopheles punctipennis*	USA
Aedes cinereus	USA	*Anopheles quadrimaculatus*	USA
Aedes excrucians	USA	*Anopheles sinensis*	China
Aedes fijensis	Fiji	*Anopheles tesellatus*	Philippines
Aedes fitchii	USA	*Anopheles walkeri*	USA
Aedes geniculatus	Europe	*Armigeres subalbatus*	Taiwan
Aedes guamensis	Guam	*Coquillettida perturbans*	USA
Aedes infirmatus	USA	*Culex anulorostris*	Guam, Fiji, Oceana
Aedes koreicus	China	*Culex bitaeniorhyncus*	Philippines
Aedes notoscriptus	Australia	*Culex declarator*	Brazil (*)
Aedes pandani	Guam	*Culex erraticus*	USA
Aedes pempaensis	Africa	*Culex gelidus*	Philippines
Aedes poecilus	Philippines	*Culex pipiens*	USA, Switzerland, Italy
Aedes polynesiensis	French Polynesia, Fiji, Samoa	*Culex pipiens quinquefasciatus*	Australia, Philippines, USA, Fiji, Japan, Taiwan, Brazil, Guam, Oceana, Africa, Singapore
Aedes pseudoscutellaris	Fiji		
Aedes punctor	Europe		
Aedes samoanus	Samoa	*Culex pipiens molestus*	UK
Aedes scapularis	Brazil	*Culex pipiens pallens*	Japan, China
Aedes sierrensis	USA	*Culex restuans*	USA
Aedes sollicitans	USA	*Culex saltanensis*	Brazil (*)
Aedes sticticus	USA	*Culex sitiens*	Guam
Aedes stimulans	USA	*Culex tarsalis*	USA
Aedes taeniorhyncus	USA, Brazil, Guyana	*Culex territans*	USA
Aedes togoi	Japan, Taiwan, Thailand	*Culex tritaeniorhynchus*	Japan, China, Malaysia
		Culex tritaeniorhynchus summorosus	Philippines
Aedes triseriatus	USA		
Aedes trivittatus	USA	*Mansonia annulata*	Malaysia
Aedes vexans	USA, Switzerland	*Mansonia bonneae*	Malaysia
Aedes vigilax	Australia	*Mansonia dives*	Malaysia
Aedes zoosophus	USA	*Mansonia Indiana*	Malaysia
Anopheles bradleyi	USA	*Mansonia titillans*	Argentina
Anopheles crucians	USA	*Mansonia uniformis*	Singapore, Philippines
Anopheles earlei	USA	*Wyeomyia bourrouli*	Brazil (*)
Anopheles francisoi	Philippines		

(*) larvae isolated at non-infective stage; (**) suspected vector but larvae not isolated from mosquito

Further reading

INTRODUCTION

Estrada-Pena A (2001) Forecasting habitat suitability for ticks and prevention of tick-borne diseases. *Veterinary Parasitology* 98, 111–132.

Patz JA, Reisen WK (2001) Immunology, climate change and vector-borne disease. *Trends in Immunology* 22, 171–172.

Shaw SE, Lerga AI, Williams S, Beugnet F, Birtles RJ, Day MJ, Kenny MJ (2003) Review of exotic infectious diseases in small animals entering the United Kingdom from abroad diagnosed by PCR. *Veterinary Record* 152, 176–177.

Woolhouse MEJ (2002) Population biology of emerging and re-emerging pathogens. *Trends in Microbiology* 10, S3–S7.

Zuckerman JN (2002) Travel medicine. *British Medical Journal* 325, 260–264.

CHAPTER 1

Baker AS (1999) Mites and ticks of domestic dnimals. *An Identification Guide and Information Source*. Natural History Museum, London.

Dryden MW, Rust MK (1994) The cat flea: biology, ecology and control. *Veterinary Parasitology* 52, 1–19.

Hoogstraal H (1966) Ticks in relation to human diseases caused by viruses. *Annual Review of Entomology* 11, 261–308.

Hoogstraal H (1967) Ticks in relation to human diseases caused by *Rickettsia* species. *Annual Review of Entomology* 12, 377–420.

Lane RP, Crosskey RW (1993) *Medical Insects and Arachnids*. Chapman & Hall, London.

Mullen G, Durden L (2002) *Medical and Veterinary Entomology*. Academic Press, Amsterdam.

Needham GR, Teal PD (1991) Off-host physiological ecology of ixodid ticks. *Annual Review of Entomology* 36, 659–681.

Wall R, Shearer D (2001) *Veterinary Ectoparasites: Biology, Pathology and Control*. 2nd edn. Blackwell Science, Oxford.

Walker A (1994) *The Arthropods of Humans and Domestic Animals*. Chapman & Hall, London.

Zumpt F (1965) *Myiasis in Man and Animals in the Old World*. Butterworths, London.

CHAPTER 2

Fenner F, Ratcliffe FN (1965) *Myxomatosis*. Cambridge University Press, Cambridge.

Hudson PJ, Rizzoli A, Grenfell BT, Heesterbeek H, Doson AP (2002) (eds) *The Ecology of Wildlife Diseases*. Oxford University Press, Oxford.

Jones CG, Ostfeld RS, Richard MP, Schauber EM, Wolff JO (1998) Chain reactions linking acorns to gypsy moth outbreaks and Lyme disease risk. *Science* 279, 1023–1026.

Perkins SE, Cattadori IM, Tagliapietra V, Rizzoli AP, Hudson PJ (2003) Empirical evidence for key hosts in persistence of a tick-borne disease. *International Journal of Parasitology* 33, 909–917.

Randolph SE, Gern L, Nuttall PA (1996) Co-feeding ticks: epidemiological significance for tick-borne pathogen transmission. *Parasitology Today* 12, 472–479.

Randolph SE, Miklisova D, Lysy J, Rogers DJ, Labuda M (1999) Incidence from co-incidence: patterns of tick infestations on rodents facilitate transmission of tick-borne encephalitis virus. *Parasitology* 118, 177–186.

Sonenshine DE, Mather TN (1994) (eds) *Ecological Dynamics of Tick-borne Zoonoses*. Oxford University Press, New York.

Williams ES, Barker IK (2001) (eds) *Infectious Diseases of Wild Mammals*. 3rd edn. Iowa State University Press, Ames.

CHAPTER 3

Gillespie RD, Mbow ML, Titus RG (2000) The immunomodulatory factors of blood feeding arthropod saliva. *Parasite Immunology* 22, 319–331.

Jittapalapong S, Stich RW, Gordon JC, Wittum TE, Barriga OO (2000) Performance of female *Rhipicephalus sanguineus* fed on dogs exposed to multiple infestations or immunization with tick salivary gland or midgut tissues. *Journal of Medical Entomology* 37, 601–611.

Kamhawi S (2000) The biological and immunomodulatory properties of sandfly saliva and its role in the establishment of *Leishmania* infections. *Microbes and Infection* 2, 1765–1773.

Matsumoto K, Inokuma H, Ohno K, Onishi T (2001) Effects of salivary gland extract from *Rhipicephalus sanguineus* on immunoglobulin class productivity of canine peripheral blood lymphocytes. *Journal of Veterinary Medical Science* 63, 325–328.

Shaw SE, Day MJ, Birtles RJ, Breitschwerdt EB (2001) Tick-borne infectious diseases of dogs. *Trends in Parasitology* 17, 74–80.

Szabo MPJ, Bechara GH (1999) Sequential histopathology at the *Rhipicephalus sanguineus* tick feeding site on dogs and guinea pigs. *Experimental and Applied Acarology* **23**, 915–928.

Wikel SK (1999) Tick modulation of host immunity: an important factor in pathogen transmission. *International Journal for Parasitology* **29**, 851–859.

Wikel SK, Alarcon-Chaidez FJ (2001) Progress towards molecular characterization of ectoparasite modulation of host immunity. *Veterinary Parasitology* **101**, 275–287.

Willadsen P (2001) The molecular revolution in the development of vaccines against ectoparasites. *Veterinary Parasitology* **101**, 353–367.

Willadsen P, Jongejan F (1999) Immunology of the tick–host interaction and the control of ticks and tick-borne diseases. *Parasitology Today* **15**, 258–262.

CHAPTER 4

Attar ZJ, Chance ML, el-Safi S, Carney J, Azazy A, El-Hadi M, Dourado C, Hommel M (2001) Latex agglutination test for the detection of urinary antigens in visceral leishmaniasis. *Acta Tropica* **15**, 11–16.

Brown SL, Hansen SL, Langone JJ (1999) Role of serology in the diagnosis of Lyme disease. *Journal of the American Medical Association* **7**, 62–66.

Courtney CH, Zeng Q (2001) Comparison of heartworm antigen test kit performance in dogs having low heartworm burdens. *Veterinary Parasitology* **96**, 317–322.

Dumler S, Aguero-Rosenfild ME (2000) Microbiology and laboratory diagnosis of tick-borne disease. In: *Tick-borne Infectious Diseases, Diagnosis and Management.* (ed BA Cunha) Marcel Dekker Inc., New York, pp. 15–54.

Gurtler RE, Cecere MC, Castanera MB, Canale D, Lauricella MA, Chuit R, Cohen JE, Segura EL (1996) Probability of infection with *Trypanosoma cruzi* of the vector *Triatoma infestans* fed on infected humans and dogs in north-west Argentina. *American Journal of Hygiene and Tropical Medicine* **55**, 24–31.

Houpikian P, Raoult D (2002) Diagnostic methods: current best practices and guidelines for identification of difficult-to-culture pathogens in infective endocarditis. *Infectious Disease Clinics of North America* **16**, 377–392.

Iqbal J, Hira PR, Saroj G, Philip R, Al-Ali F, Madda PJ, Sher A (2002) Imported visceral leishmaniasis: diagnostic dilemmas and comparative analysis of three assays. *Journal of Clinical Microbiology* **40**, 475–479.

La Scola B, Raoult D (1999) Culture of *Bartonella quintana* and *Bartonella henselae* from human samples: a 5-year experience (1993–1998). *Journal of Clinical Microbiology* **37**, 1899–1905.

Paek SH, Lee SH, Cho JH, Kim YS (2000) Development of rapid one-step immunochromatographic assay. *Methods* **22**, 53–60.

Persing DH (1996) *PCR Protocols for Emerging Infectious Diseases.* American Society for Microbiology Press, Washington.

Smits HL, Chee HD, Eapen CK, Kuriakose M, Sugathan S, Gasem MH, Yersin C, Sakasi D, Lai-A-Fat RF, Hartskeerl RA, Liesdek B, Abdoel TH, Goris MG, Gussenhoven GC (2001) Latex-based, rapid and easy assay for human leptospirosis in a single test format. *Tropical Medicine and International Health* **6**, 114–118.

Zarlenga DS, Higgins J (2001) PCR as a diagnostic and quantitative technique in veterinary parasitology. *Veterinary Parasitology* **22**, 215–230.

CHAPTER 5

Bredal WP, Gjerde B, Eberhard ML, Aleksandersen M, Wilhelmsen DK, Mansfield LS (1998) Adult *Dirofilaria repens* in a subcutaneous granuloma on the chest of a dog. *Journal of Small Animal Practice* **39**, 595–597.

Courtney CH, Zeng QY (2001) Comparison of heartworm antigen test kit performance in dogs having low heartworm burdens. *Veterinary Parasitology* **96**, 317–322.

DeFrancesco TC, Atkins CE, Miller MW, Meurs KM, Keene BW (2001) Use of echocardiography for the diagnosis of heartworm disease in cats: 43 cases (1985–1997). *Journal of the American Veterinary Medical Association* **218**, 66–69.

Goodwin JK (1998) The serological diagnosis of heartworm infection in dogs and cats. *Clinical Techniques in Small Animal Practice* **13**, 83–87.

Kittleson M (1999) Heartworm infestation and disease (dirofilariasis). In: *Small Animal Cardiovascular Medicine.* (eds MD Kittleson and RD Kienle) Mosby, St. Louis, pp. 370–401.

Knauer KW (1998) Human dirofilariasis. *Clinical Techniques in Small Animal Practice* **13**, 96–98.

Knight D (1999) Guidelines for the diagnosis, prevention and management of heartworm (*Dirofilaria immitis*) infection in dogs. http://heartwormsociety.org/ahsguide.htm

Ludlam KW, Jachowski Jr LA, Otto GF (1970) Potential vectors of *Dirofilaria immitis*. *Journal of the American Veterinary Medical Association* **157**, 1354–1359.

Miller MW (1998) Feline dirofilariasis. *Clinical Techniques in Small Animal Practice* **13**, 99–109.

Rawlings CA, Calvert CA, Glaus TM, Jacobs GJ (1994) Surgical removal of heartworms. *Seminars in Veterinary Medicine and Surgery (Small Animal)* **9**, 200–205.

Rawlings CA (2002) Effects of monthly heartworm preventatives on dogs with young heartworm infections. *Journal of the American Animal Hospital Association* **38**, 311–314.

Snyder PS, Levy JK, Salute ME, Gorman SP, Kubilis PS, Smail PW, George LL (2000) Performance of serologic tests used to detect heartworm infection in cats. *Journal of the American Veterinary Medical Association* **216**, 693–700.

Strickland KN (1998) Canine and feline caval syndrome. *Clinical Techniques in Small Animal Practice* **13**, 88–95.

CHAPTER 6

Babesiosis

Camacho AT, Pallas E, Gestal JJ, Guitian FJ, Olmeda AS, Goethert HK, Telford SR (2001) Infection of dogs in north-west Spain with a *Babesia microti*-like agent. *Veterinary Record* **149**, 552–555.

Carret C, Walas F, Carcy B, Grande N, Precigout E, Moubri K, Schetters TP, Gorenflot A (1999) *Babesia canis canis, Babesia canis vogeli, Babesia canis rossi*: differentiation of the three subspecies by a restriction fragment length polymorphism analysis on amplified small subunit ribosomal RNA genes. *Journal of Eukaryote Microbiology* **46**, 298–303.

Homer MJ, Aguilar-Delfin I, Telford SR, Krause PJ, Persing DH (2000) Babesiosis. *Clinical Microbiology Reviews* **13**, 451–469.

Kjemtrup AM, Kocan AA, Whitwoth L, Meinkoth J, Birkenheuer AJ, Cummings J, Boudreaux MK, Stockham SL, Irizarry-Rovira A, Conrad PA (2000) There are at least three genetically distinct small piroplasms from dogs. *International Journal for Parasitology* **30**, 1501–1505.

Jacobson LS, Swan GE (1995) Supportive treatment of canine babesiosis. *Journal of the South African Veterinary Association* **66**, 95–105.

Melhorn H, Walldorf V (1988) Life cycles. In: *Parasitology in Focus: Facts and Trends.* (ed H Melhorn) Springer-Verlag, Berlin, pp. 1–148.

Schoeman T, Lobetti RG, Jacobson LS, Penzhorn BL (2001) Feline babesiosis: signalment, clinical pathology and concurrent infections. *Journal of the South African Veterinary Association* **72**, 4–11.

Yamane I, Conrad PA, Gardner I (1993) *Babesia gibsoni* infections in dogs. *Journal of Protozoology* **3**, 111–125.

Zahler M, Schein E, Rinder H, Gothe R (1998) Characteristic genotypes discriminate between *Babesia canis* isolates of differing vector specificity and pathogenicity to dogs. *Parasitology Research* **84**, 544–548.

Zahler M, Rinder H, Schein E, Gothe R (2000) Detection of new pathogenic *Babesia microti*-like species in dogs. *Veterinary Parasitology* **89**, 241–248.

Cytauxzoonosis

Meinkoth J, Kocan AA, Whitworth L, Murphy G, Fox CJ, Woods JP (2000) Cats surviving natural infection with *Cytauxzoon felis*: 18 cases (1997–1998). *Journal of Veterinary Internal Medicine* **14**, 521–525.

CHAPTER 7

Baneth G, Weigler B (1997) A retrospective case-control study of canine hepatozoonosis in Israel. *Journal of Veterinary Internal Medicine* **11**, 1891–1894.

Baneth G, Aroch I, Tal N, Harrus S (1998) *Hepatozoon* species infection in domestic cats: a retrospective study. *Veterinary Parasitology* **79**, 123–133.

Baneth G, Barta JR, Shkap V, Martin DS, Macintire DK, Vincent-Johnson N (2000) Genetic and antigenic evidence supports the separation of *Hepatozoon canis* and *Hepatozoon americanum* at the species level. *Journal of Clinical Microbiology* **38**, 1298–1301.

Baneth G, Samish M, Aroch I, Alekseev Y, Shkap V (2001) Transmission of *Hepatozoon canis* to dogs by naturally fed or percutaneously injected *Rhipicephalus sanguineus* ticks. *Journal of Parasitology* **87**, 606–611.

Baneth G, Mathew JS, Shkap V, McIntire DK, Barta JR, Ewing SA (2003) Canine hepatozoonosis: two diseases caused by separate *Hepatozoon* species. *Trends in Parasitology* **19**, 27–31.

Ewing SA, Panciera RJ, Mathew JS, Cummings CA, Kocan AA (2000) American canine hepatozoonosis: an emerging disease in the New World. *Annals of the New York Academy of Sciences* **916**, 81–92.

Macintire DK, Vincent-Johnson NA, Kane CW, Lindsay DS, Blagburn BL, Dillon AR (2001) Treatment of dogs infected with *Hepatozoon americanum*: 53 cases (1989–1998). *Journal of the American Veterinary Medical Association* **218**, 77–82.

Mathew JS, Ewing SA, Panciera RJ, Woods JP (1998) Experimental transmission of *Hepatozoon americanum* to dogs by the Gulf Coast tick, *Amblyomma maculatum*. *Veterinary Parasitology* **80**, 1–14.

Panciera RJ, Ewing SA, Mathew JS, Lebenbauer TW, Cummings CA, Woods JP (1999) Canine hepatozoonosis: comparison of lesions and parasites in skeletal muscle of dogs experimentally or naturally infected with *Hepatozoon americanum*. *Veterinary Parasitology* **82**, 261–272.

Vincent-Johnson NA, Macintire DK, Lindsay DS, Lenz SD, Baneth G, Shkap V, Blagburn BL (1997) A new *Hepatozoon* species from dogs: description of the causative agent of canine hepatozoonosis in North America. *Journal of Parasitology* **83**, 1165–1172.

CHAPTER 8

Baneth G, Shaw SE (2002) Chemotherapy of canine leishmaniasis. *Veterinary Parasitology* **106**, 315–324.

Ciaramella P, Oliva G, de Luna R, Gradoni L, Ambrosio R, Cortese L, Scalone A, Persechino A, De Luna R (1997) A retrospective clinical study of canine leishmaniasis in 150 dogs naturally infected by *Leishmania infantum*. *Veterinary Record* **141**, 539–543.

GarciaAlonso M, Blanco A, Reina D, Serrano FJ, Alonso C, Nieto CG (1996) Immunopathology of the uveitis in canine leishmaniasis. *Parasite Immunology* **18**, 617–623.

Gradoni L (2001) An update on anti-leishmanial vaccine candidates and prospects for a canine *Leishmania* vaccine. *Veterinary Parasitology* **100**, 87–103.

Koutinas AF, Polizopoulou ZS, Saridomichelakis MN, Argyriadis D, Fytianou A, Plevraki KG (1999) Clinical considerations on canine visceral leishmaniasis in Greece: a retrospective study of 158 cases (1989–1996). *Journal of the American Animal Hospital Association* 35, 376–383.

Koutinas AF, Scott DW, Kantos V, Lekkas S (1993) Skin lesions in canine leishmaniasis (Kala-Azar): a clinical and histopathological study on 22 spontaneous cases in Greece. *Veterinary Dermatology* 3, 121–131.

Nieto CG, Navarrete I, Habela MA, Serrano F, Redondo E (1992) Pathological changes in kidneys of dogs with natural *Leishmania* infection. *Veterinary Parasitology* 45, 33–47.

Pena MT, Roura X, Davidson MG (2000) Ocular and periocular manifestations of leishmaniasis in dogs: 105 cases (1993–1998). *Veterinary Ophthalmology* 3, 35–41.

Pinelli E, Killick-Kendrick R, Wagenaar J, Bernadina W, Del Real G, Ruitenberg J (1994) Cellular and humoral immune responses in dogs experimentally and naturally infected with *Leishmania infantum*. *Infection and Immunity* 62, 229–235.

Quinnell RJ, Courtney O, Davidson S, Garcez L, Lambson B, Ramos P, Shaw JJ, Shaw MA, Dye C (2001) Detection of *Leishmania infantum* by PCR, serology and cellular immune response in a cohort study of Brazilian dogs. *Parasitology* 122, 253–261.

Solano-Gallego L, Llull J, Ramos G, Riera C, Arboix M, Alberola J, Ferrer L (2000) The Ibizian Hound presents a predominantly cellular immune response against natural *Leishmania* infection. *Veterinary Parasitology* 90, 37–45.

Solano-Gallego L, Morell P, Arboix M, Alberola J, Ferrer L (2001) Prevalence of *Leishmania infantum* infection in dogs living in an area of canine leishmaniasis endemicity using PCR on several tissues and serology. *Journal of Clinical Microbiology* 39, 560–563.

CHAPTER 9

Appel MJG, Allan S, Jacobson RH, Lauderdale TL, Chang YF, Shin SJ, Thomford JW, Todhunter RJ, Summers BA (1993) Experimental Lyme disease in dogs produces arthritis and persistent infection. *Journal of Infectious Diseases* 167, 651–664.

Azuma Y, Isogai E, Isogai H, Kawamura K (1994) Canine Lyme disease: clinical and serological evaluations in 21 dogs in Japan. *Veterinary Record* 134, 369–372.

Chang YF, Straubinger RK, Jacobson RH, Kim JB, Kim TJ, Kim D, Shin SJ, Appel MJG (1996) Dissemination of *Borrelia burgdorferi* after experimental infection in dogs. *Journal of Spirochetal Tick-Borne Disease* 3, 80–86.

Dambach DM, Smith CA, Lewis RM, Van Winkle TJ (1997) Morphologic, immunohistochemical and ultrastructural characterization of a distinctive renal lesion in dogs putatively associated with *Borrelia burgdorferi* infection: 49 cases (1987–1992). *Veterinary Pathology* 34, 85–96.

Hovius KE, Stark LAM, Bleumink-Pluym NMC, Van der Pol I, Verbeek-De Kruif N, Rijpkema SGT, Schouls LM, Houwers DJ (1999) Presence and distribution of *Borrelia burgdorferi sensu lato* in internal organs and skin of naturally infected symptomatic and asymptomatic dogs, as detected by polymerase chain reaction. *Veterinary Quarterly* 21, 54–58.

Hovius JWR, Hovius KE, Oei A, Houwers DJ, Van Dam AP (2000) Antibodies against specific proteins of, and immobilizing activity against, three strains of *Borrelia burgdorferi sensu lato* can be found in symptomatic but not in infected asymptomatic dogs. *Journal of Clinical Microbiology* 38, 2611–2621.

Kornblatt AN, Urband PH, Steere AC (1985) Arthritis caused by *Borrelia burgdorferi* in dogs. *Journal of the American Veterinary Medical Association* 186, 960–964.

Levy SA, Duray PH (1988) Complete heart block in a dog seropositive for *Borrelia burgdorferi*. *Journal of Veterinary Internal Medicine* 2, 138–144.

Magnarelli LA, Anderson JF, Kaufmann AF, Liebermann LL, Whitney GD (1985) Borreliosis in dogs from southern Connecticut. *Journal of the American Veterinary Medical Association* 186, 955–959.

Straubinger RK, Straubinger AF, Härter L, Jacobson RH, Chang YF, Summers BA, Erb HN, Appel MJG (1997) *Borrelia burgdorferi* migrates into joint capsules and causes an up-regulation of interleukin-8 in synovial membranes of dogs experimentally infected with ticks. *Infection and Immunity* 65, 1273–1285.

Straubinger RK (2000) PCR-based quantification of *Borrelia burgdorferi* organisms in canine tissues over a 500-day postinfection period. *Journal of Clinical Microbiology* 38, 2191–2199.

CHAPTER 10

Birtles RJ, Laycock G, Kenny MJ, Shaw SE, Day MJ (2002) Prevalence of *Bartonella* species causing bacteraemia in domesticated and companion animals in the United Kingdom. *Veterinary Record* 151, 225–229.

Breitschwerdt EB, Atkins CE, Brown TT, Kordick DL, Snyder PS (1999) *Bartonella vinsonii* subsp. *berkhoffii* and related members of the alpha subdivision of the Proteobacteria in dogs with cardiac arrhythmias, endocarditis or myocarditis. *Journal of Clinical Microbiology* 37, 3618–3626.

Breitschwerdt EB, Kordick DL (2000) *Bartonella* infection in animals: carriership, reservoir potential, pathogenicity and zoonotic potential for human infection. *Clinical Microbiology Reviews* 13, 428–438.

Chomel BB, Kasten RW, Sykes JE, Boulouis HJ, Breitschwerdt EB (2003) Clinical impact of persistent *Bartonella* bacteremia in humans and animals. *Annals of the New York Academy of Science* 990, 267–278.

Guptill L, Slater L, Wu CC, Lin TL, Glickman LT, Welch DF, HogenEsch H (1997) Experimental infection of young specific pathogen-free cats with *Bartonella henselae*. *Journal of Infectious Diseases* 176, 206–216.

Kitchell BE, Fan TM, Kordick D, Breitschwerdt EB, Wollenberg G, Lichtensteiger CA (2000) Peliosis hepatis in a dog infected with *Bartonella henselae*. *Journal of the American Veterinary Medical Association* **216**, 519–523.

Kordick DL, Brown TT, Shin K, Breitschwerdt EB (1999) Clinical and pathologic evaluation of chronic *Bartonella henselae* or *Bartonella clarridgeiae* infection in cats. *Journal of Clinical Microbiology* **37**, 1536–1547.

Pappalardo BL, Brown TT, Tompkins M, Breitschwerdt EB (2001) Immunopathology of *Bartonella vinsonii* (*berkhoffii*) in experimentally infected dogs. *Veterinary Immunology and Immunopathology* **83**, 125–147.

Pappalardo BL, Brown T, Gookin JL, Morrill CL, Breitschwerdt EB (2000) Granulomatous disease associated with *Bartonella* infection in two dogs. *Journal of Veterinary Internal Medicine* **14**, 37–42.

Mexas AM, Hancock SI, Breitschwerdt EB (2002) *Bartonella henselae* and *Bartonella elizabethae* as potential canine pathogens. *Journal of Clinical Microbiology* **40**, 4670–4674.

CHAPTER 11

E. canis

Dawson JE, Ewing SA (1992) Susceptibility of dogs to infection with *Ehrlichia chaffeensis*, causative agent of human ehrlichiosis. *American Journal of Veterinary Research* **53**, 1322–1327.

Dumler JS, Walker DH (2001) Tick-borne ehrlichioses. *Lancet Infectious Diseases* **April**, 21–28.

Harrus S, Waner T, Bark H (1997) Canine monocytic ehrlichiosis: an update. *Compendium on Continuing Education for the Practicing Veterinarian* **19**, 431–447.

Harrus S, Waner T, Bark H, Jongejan F, Cornelissen AWC (1999) Canine monocytic ehrlichiosis: recent advances. *Journal of Clinical Microbiology* **37**, 2745–2749.

Kelly PJ (2000) Canine ehrlichioses: an update. *Journal of the South African Veterinary Association* **71**, 77–86.

Murphy GL, Ewing SA, Whitworth LC, Fox JC, Kocan AA (1998) A molecular and serologic survey of *Ehrlichia canis* and *E. ewingii* in dogs and ticks from Oklahoma. *Veterinary Parasitology* **79**, 325–339.

Neer TM (1998) Ehrlichiosis. Canine monocytic and granulocytic ehrlichiosis. In: *Infectious Diseases of the Dog and Cat*. (ed CE Greene) WB Saunders, Philadelphia, pp. 139–154.

Ristic M, Holland CJ (1993) Canine ehrlichiosis. In: *Rickettsial and Chlamydial Diseases of Domestic Animals*. (eds Z Woldehiwet and M Ristic) Pergamon Press, New York, pp. 169–186.

Stubbs CJ, Holland CJ, Reif JS, Wheeler S, Bruns C, Lappin MR (2000) Feline ehrlichiosis. *Compendium on Continuing Education for the Practicing Veterinarian* **22**, 307–317.

Waner T, Harrus S, Jongejan F, Bark H, Keysary A, Cornelissen WCA (2001) Significance of serological testing for ehrlichial diseases in dogs with special emphasis on the diagnosis of canine monocytic ehrlichiosis caused by *Ehrlichia canis*. *Veterinary Parasitology* **95**, 1–15.

A. phagocytophilum

Bakken JS, Dumler JS (2000) Human granulocytic ehrlichiosis. *Clinical Infectious Diseases* **31**, 554–560.

Egenvall A, Björersdorff A, Lilliehöök I, Olsson Engvall E, Karlstam E, Artursson K, Hedhammar Å, Gunnarsson A (1998) Early manifestations of granulocytic ehrlichiosis in dogs inoculated experimentally with a Swedish *Ehrlichia* species isolate. *Veterinary Record* **143**, 412–417.

Egenvall A, Bonnett BN, Gunnarsson A, Hedhammar Å, Shoukri M, Bornstein S, Artursson K (2000) Seroprevalence of granulocytic *Ehrlichia* spp. and *Borrelia burgdorferi sensu lato* in Swedish dogs 1991–1994. *Scandinavian Journal of Infectious Diseases* **32**, 19–25.

Egenvall A, Lilliehook I, Bjoersdorff A, Engvall EO, Karlstam E, Artursson K, Heldtander M, Gunnarsson A (2000) Detection of granulocytic *Ehrlichia* species DNA by PCR in persistently infected dogs. *Veterinary Record* **146**, 186–190.

Herron MJ, Nelson CM, Larson J, Snapp KR, Kansas GS, Goodman JL (2000) Intracellular parasitism by the human granulocytic ehrlichiosis bacterium through the P-selectin ligand, PSGL-1. *Science* **288**, 1653–1656.

Lepidi H, Bunnell JE, Martin ME, Madigan JE, Stuen S, Dumler JS (2000) Comparative pathology and immunohistology associated with clinical illness after *Ehrlichia phagocytophila*-group infections. *American Journal of Tropical Medicine and Hygiene* **62**, 29–37.

Levin ML, Fish D (2000) Acquisition of co-infection and simultaneous transmission of *Borrelia burgdorferi* and *Ehrlichia phagocytophila* by *Ixodes scapularis* ticks. *Infection and Immunity* **68**, 2183–2186.

Lilliehöök I, Egenvall A, Tvedten HW (1998) Hematopathology in dogs experimentally infected with a Swedish granulocytic *Ehrlichia* species. *Veterinary Clinical Pathology* **27**, 116–122.

Walker DH (2000) The Task Force on consensus approach for ehrlichiosis. Diagnosing human ehrlichiosis: current status and recommendations. *American Society of Microbiology News* **66**, 287–290.

Zeidner NS, Burkot TR, Massung RF, Nicholson WL, Dolan MC, Rutherford JS, Biggerstaff BJ, Maupin GO (2000) Transmission of the agent of human granulocytic ehrlichiosis by *Ixodes spinipalpis* ticks: evidence of an enzootic cycle of dual infection with *Borrelia burgdorferi* in northern Colorado. *Journal of Infectious Diseases* **182**, 616–619.

A. platys

Harrus S, Aroch I, Lavy E, Bark H (1997) Clinical manifestations of infectious canine cyclic thrombocytopenia. *Veterinary Record* **141**, 247–250.

deAlvarado CMA, Parra OD, Palmar M, Chango RE, Alvarado MC (1997) *Ehrlichia platys*: antigen processing and use of the indirect fluorescent antibody test (IFA) in canines and humans. *Revista Cientifica-Facultad de Ciencias Veterinarias* **2**, 99–109.

Chang ACH, Chang WL, Lin CT, Pan MJ, Lee SC (1996) Canine infectious cyclic thrombocytopenia found in Taiwan. *Journal of Veterinary Medical Science* **58**, 473–476.

Brown GK, Martin AR, Roberts TK, Aitkin RJ (2001) Detection of *Ehrlichia platys* in dogs in Australia. *Australian Veterinary Journal* **79**, 554–558.

CHAPTER 12

Bouyer DH, Stenos J, Crocquet-Valdes P, Moron CG (2001) *Rickettsia felis*: molecular characterization of a new member of the spotted fever group. *International Journal of Systematic and Evolutionary Microbiology* **51**, 339–341.

Breitschwerdt EB, Papich MG, Hegarty BC, Gilger B, Hancock SI, Davidson MG (1999) Efficacy of doxycycline, azithromycin or trovafloxacin for treatment of experimental Rocky Mountain spotted fever in dogs. *Antimicrobial Agents and Chemotherapy* **43**, 813–821.

Breitschwerdt EB, Walker DH, Levy MG, Burgdorfer W, Corbett WT, Hurlbert SA, Stebbins ME, Curtis BC, Allen DA (1988) Clinical, hematologic and humoral immune response in female dogs inoculated with *Rickettsia rickettsii* and *Rickettsia montana*. *American Journal of Veterinary Research* **49**, 70–76.

Gasser AM, Birkenheuer AJ, Breitschwerdt EB (2001) Canine Rocky Mountain spotted fever: a retrospective study of 30 cases. *Journal of the American Animal Hospital Association* **37**, 41–48.

Greene CE, Burgdorfer W, Cavagnolo R, Philip RN, Peacock MG (1985) Rocky Mountain spotted fever in dogs and its differentiation from canine ehrlichiosis. *Journal of the American Veterinary Medical Association* **186**, 465–472.

Greene CE, Marks MA, Lappin MR, Breitschwerdt EB, Wolski NA, Burgdorfer W (1993) Comparison of latex agglutination, indirect immunofluorescent antibody and enzyme immunoassay methods for serodiagnosis of Rocky Mountain spotted fever in dogs. *American Journal of Veterinary Research* **54**, 20–28.

Holman RC, Paddock CD, Curns AT, Krebs JW, McQuiston JH, Childs JE (2001) Analysis of risk factors for fatal Rocky Mountain spotted fever: evidence for superiority of tetracyclines for therapy. *Journal of Infectious Diseases* **184**, 1437–1444.

Sexton DJ, Kanj SS, Wilson K, Cory GR, Hegarty BC, Levy MG, Brietschwerdt EB (1994) The use of a polymerase chain reaction as a diagnostic test for Rocky Mountain spotted fever. *American Journal of Tropical Medicine and Hygiene* **50**, 59–63.

Sorvillo FJ, Gondo B, Emmons R, Ryan P, Waterman SH, Tilzer A, Andersen EM, Murray RA, Barr AR (1993) A suburban focus of endemic typhus in Los Angeles County: association with seropositive cats and opossums. *American Journal of Tropical Medicine and Hygiene* **48**, 269–273.

Weiser IB, Greene CE (1989) Dermal necrosis associated with Rocky Mountain spotted fever in four dogs. *Journal of the American Veterinary Medical Association* **195**, 1756–1758.

CHAPTER 13

Barr SC (1991) Canine American trypanosomiasis. *Compendium on Continuing Education for the Practicing Veterinarian* **13**, 745–754.

Carlson ME (1996) *Yersinia pestis* infection in cats. *Feline Practice* **24**, 22–24.

Eidson M, Elstad JP, Rollag OJ (1991) Clinical, clinicopathological and pathologic features of plague in cats: 119 cases (1977–1985). *Journal of the American Veterinary Medical Association* **199**, 1191–1196

Lichtensteiger CA, Heinz-Taheny K, Osborne TS, Novak RJ, Lewis BA, Firth ML (2003) West Nile virus encephalitis and myocarditis in wolf and dog. *Journal of Emerging Infectious Diseases* **9**, 1303–1306.

Morita C, Katsuyama J, Yanase T, Ueno H, Muramatsu Y, Hohdatsu T, Koyama H (1994) Seroepidemiological survey of *Coxiella burnetii* in domestic cats in Japan. *Microbiology and Immunology* **38**, 1001–1003.

Nagaoka H, Sugieda M, Akiyama M, Nishina T, Akahane S, Fujiwara K (1998) Isolation of *Coxiella burnetii* from the vagina of feline clients at veterinary clinics. *Journal of Veterinary Medical Science* **60**, 251–252.

Reid HW (1998) Louping ill. In: *Infectious Diseases of the Dog and Cat.* (ed CE Greene) WB Saunders, Philadelphia, pp. 133–134.

Shaw SE, Birtles RJ, Day MJ (2001) Arthropod-transmitted infectious diseases of cats. *Journal of Feline Medicine and Surgery* **3**, 193–209.

Weissenbock H, Holzmann H (1997) Tick-borne encephalitis in Austrian dogs. *Veterinary Record* **139**, 575–576.

Woods JP, Crystal MA, Morton RW, Panciera RJ (1998) Tularemia in two cats. *Journal of the American Animal Hospital Association* **212**, 81–85.

Index